The

Emerging

HEALTHCARE

LEADER

LAURIE BAEDKE

NATALIE LAMBERTON

The

Emerging
HEALTHCARE
LEADER

Second
Edition

A Field Guide

ACHE Management Series

Your board, staff, or clients may also benefit from this book's insight. For information on quantity discounts, contact the Health Administration Press Marketing Manager at (312) 424-9450.

This publication is intended to provide accurate and authoritative information in regard to the subject matter covered. It is sold, or otherwise provided, with the understanding that the publisher is not engaged in rendering professional services. If professional advice or other expert assistance is required, the services of a competent professional should be sought.

The statements and opinions contained in this book are strictly those of the authors and do not represent the official positions of the American College of Healthcare Executives or the Foundation of the American College of Healthcare Executives.

22   5 4 3

Library of Congress Cataloging-in-Publication Data
Names: Baedke, Laurie, author. | Lamberton, Natalie, author.
Title: The emerging healthcare leader : a field guide / Laurie Baedke and
    Natalie Lamberton.
Description: Second edition. | Chicago, IL : Health Administration Press,
    [2018] | Series: HAP/ACHE management series | Includes bibliographical
    references.
Identifiers: LCCN 2018000504 (print) | LCCN 2018000943 (ebook) | ISBN
    9781567939910 (ebook) | ISBN 9781567939927 (xml) | ISBN 9781567939934
    (epub) | ISBN 9781567939941 (mobi) | ISBN 9781567939903 (alk. paper)
Subjects: LCSH: Health care teams—Management. | Health services
    administrators—Vocational guidance. | Health services administration.
Classification: LCC R729.5.H4 (ebook) | LCC R729.5.H4 B34 2018 (print) | DDC
    362.1068—dc23
LC record available at https://lccn.loc.gov/2018000504

The paper used in this publication meets the minimum requirements of American National Standard for Information Sciences—Permanence of Paper for Printed Library Materials, ANSI Z39.48-1984. ∞ ™

Acquisitions editor: Janet Davis; Manuscript editor: Sharon Sofinski; Project manager: Andrew Baumann; Cover designer: Marisa Jackson; Layout: PerfecType

Found an error or a typo? We want to know! Please e-mail it to hapbooks@ache.org, mentioning the book's title and putting "Book Error" in the subject line.

For photocopying and copyright information, please contact Copyright Clearance Center at www.copyright.com or (978) 750-8400.

Health Administration Press
A division of the Foundation of the American
    College of Healthcare Executives
300 S. Riverside Plaza, Suite 1900
Chicago, IL 60606-6698
(312) 424-2800

To my husband, Wes, and our beautiful children, Sophia and Quinn. This book could not have happened without your patience and encouragement. I love you.

To my mom, for instilling a passion for learning, and my dad, for modeling a tireless drive and pursuit of excellence. Thank you.

To those who have mentored me and shared so generously of their wisdom and experience, I am forever in your debt and pay it forward.

To Natalie, thank you for your partnership on this journey. You are an amazing woman and I am blessed to call you friend.

—Laurie

To my mom and dad, for teaching me to always do my best.

To my siblings, Nicole and Newman, for being my best friends.

To Laurie, for bringing me along on this wonderful adventure. I've learned so much.

Last but not least, to my husband, Rory, for his unwavering support of everything I am and everything I do. Thanks for being a shining example of an authentic leader and, most important, a lifelong partner.

Much love.

—Natalie

Contents

Foreword to the First Edition

HUNDREDS OF BOOKS are available to students and the business community. Many offer incredible insights into specific best practices of running an organization. Books on leadership, management styles, lean operations, and motivating and cultivating your workforce are readily available. There is also a subset of business books that dive into the particulars of the healthcare field. Books and speakers are plentiful for those who wish to learn how to navigate the ever-changing environment that is healthcare management. What has been lacking, until now, is a guide for students that bridges the gap between their academic pursuit and their first leadership role in healthcare.

More than theory, *The Emerging Healthcare Leader: A Field Guide* is your road map for that journey. A refreshing and practical tool, this should be your handbook, your back-pocket how-to resource as you traverse the early years of your leadership career.

In their engaging and authentic style, authors Laurie Baedke and Natalie Lamberton offer valuable insight, real-world examples, and sage wisdom that many do not accumulate until decades later in their careers. Additionally, what they so courageously share is the truth that successful people often fail. While Natalie and Laurie have achieved admirable successes, positions, opportunities, and accolades, they've also stumbled and misstepped along the way. Their willingness to share those experiences so that others can learn from them is a hallmark of great leadership. Each author has a proven track record of success in her short career.

I had the pleasure of meeting Natalie as my first fellow for the Poudre Valley Health System in Fort Collins, Colorado. She was an outstanding student and employee, and I could see her passion for healthcare way back then. She keeps good company, as through her I've had the opportunity to meet and get to know Laurie at the annual Congress of the American College of Healthcare Executives, where they've both served as faculty for the perennial favorite session "Developing the Next Generation of Leaders: Lessons from the First 10 Years."

This book is an undeniably compelling body of work, born from that successful Congress session. For good reason, students flock to that session to soak up the content, which has encouraged and equipped so many early careerists in healthcare administration over the years. Brimming with practical suggestions, lessons learned, stories, and anecdotes, the book offers wisdom from which newcomers to the field and industry veterans alike can learn.

Civil leader and philosopher Mahatma Gandhi once said, "The best way to find yourself is to lose yourself in the service of others." It has been a pleasure and a privilege to observe Natalie's and Laurie's journey. Their passion for investing in emerging leaders (those just a few short steps behind them), their commitment to excellence and personal development, and their tireless enthusiasm to serve and mentor give me confidence that the next generation is in good hands. Healthcare needs great leaders—strong, humble, capable individuals who will rise to serve this profession. This book is a resource to equip them.

Rulon F. Stacey, PhD, FACHE
Chairman (2011–2012), American College of Healthcare Executives
Managing Director, Navigant Consulting

Introduction

THIS BOOK—*The Emerging Healthcare Leader: A Field Guide*—is all about you. Not your parents, not your preceptors, not the seasoned CEO whom you aspire to become. We wrote it with your healthcare career in mind and with our industry knowledge and experiences as guides. Why? Our answer is threefold.

First, we believe in the enormous contributions you can impart. Today, you may still be learning or struggling to enter healthcare. But tomorrow, you will be among the principals in the field—whether making operational and workforce decisions for a patient care unit or an entire facility, consulting with chief executives and governing boards, running a physician or clinical practice, developing and implementing national policies and standards, or teaching future leaders. Before then, you need to seek out as much advice and insight as possible to mentally and emotionally prepare yourself for the changes and challenges (and the joys) ahead. And we wish to be part—even in a small way—of your journey to get there.

Second, we are passionate about healthcare. Working in this industry—regardless of your job title—is formidable but also an awesome, rewarding privilege. We want to see the US healthcare system become the best in the world, and that can only happen if we put conscientious, well-trained, and caring people in the top positions. That starts with you. And you represent the next generation of leaders.

Third, we want to give back to the field. We are fortunate to have had countless mentors, colleagues, teachers, and superiors who graciously and generously invested time and effort in our own career development. This is why we have been so eager to return the favor by engaging graduate and undergraduate students year-round. We mentor them, review their resumes, and conduct mock interviews. Plus, we stay active and connected in the industry, an essential activity for any serious professional.

We designed the book to be a casual but an informative read—much like how we designed the early careerist sessions we present during the American College of Healthcare Executives (ACHE) Congress on Healthcare Leadership. In fact, it was the positive reception to these sessions—along with the lessons we've both accumulated over the years—that convinced us to compile our advice and recommendations in book form. We can't be more thrilled to share these with you and a larger audience of emerging leaders.

This second edition is an encore to our original text. In it, we expand the content to include two brand-new chapters on the topics of emotional intelligence and successful onboarding to new roles. We also dig a bit deeper into certain conversations and refresh the content around etiquette and social media. And, finally, we double down and add four new Notes to My 25-Year-Old Self from outstanding leaders in our industry.

WHO WE ARE

What makes us qualified to talk about career development? Like you, we were new to healthcare once, each armed only with a master's degree in health administration and a desire to be involved in something bigger than ourselves. Like you, we sought guidance from others and pursued multiple opportunities. Like you, we have worked extremely hard to get where we are today.

Laurie became a hospital vice president at age 22 and then went on to become a healthcare consultant, an executive coach, a speaker, and now a graduate program director. Natalie—after a career as a schoolteacher and a stint as a director of a hospital's retail services—became a hospital CEO at age 29 and has since served in leadership positions for a number of healthcare organizations, coming full circle as a CEO again. We realize that our results are not typical, given that senior-level positions take years to attain. But our results are examples of what's possible when you commit yourself early to personal and professional development, to building relationships (which could one day lead to tremendous opportunities), and to presenting yourself as someone who is ready for the next level.

For nine years now, we have presented a well-received early careerist session during the ACHE Congress. This is a collaboration born out of our initial meeting ten years ago and our mutual interest in widening our professional scope and contributing to the field. Individually, we seize every opportunity to learn and to share that knowledge with up-and-comers—in or out of the industry.

Our education, ongoing training, diverse experiences, civic and professional activities, and everyday work duties give us a full picture of what a young careerist needs and wants.

WHAT THE BOOK IS AND IS NOT

This book is a guide, a reference, a resource, a companion manual. But it is *not* a textbook—nor is it your boss's or CEO's management book. It is yours. So put down your highlighter, grab your coffee mug, and get comfortable.

Superb graduate and undergraduate health administration programs do an excellent job of exposing their students to management and care delivery scenarios in actual organizations. These programs even offer elective courses focused on professional decorum and skill development. And that's great!

Look at this book then as an extension of such a curriculum—and so much more. It is not stuffed with theories or academic language; instead, it is neatly packed with applicable strategies and straightforward (even amusing) examples. If you want to know what self-awareness is, for example, the book does not go on and on about the philosophy and psychology of the self. Rather, it gives you practical tips on how to become self-aware.

The content is tailored to the particular concerns or curiosities of a new healthcare graduate trying to build or expand a career, or even an established healthcare professional trying to switch disciplines, update or enhance existing skills, or learn ways to advise young protégés or students.

The 15 chapters here are divided into three parts. Part I (containing chapters 1 through 5) discusses self-awareness, self-management, and the continued development of emotional intelligence as well as the by-products of these concepts—strong character, conscious commitment, and self-discipline. These concepts are the foundation for the rest of the ideas in the book. Part II (containing chapters 6 through 11) expands the part I concepts and introduces more practices that you can adopt (or at least consider) now, including cultivating your personal brand, understanding your own leadership style, learning and rebounding from failures, creating lasting networking relationships, and mentoring. Part III (containing chapters 12 through 15) covers the nitty-gritty of pursuing internship opportunities and being an intern, mastering the interview process, successfully navigating the onboarding process in a new role, and managing your own career path.

Each chapter includes the following:

- An opening quote that represents the essence of the chapter
- Reading Points, a list of the main topics in the chapter
- Remember These, a list of the lessons learned or takeaways from the chapter

Two more features, spread throughout the book, are worth mentioning:

- Rookie Mistakes, a sidebar of don'ts. We (and some of our colleagues) have made mistakes—lots of them—throughout our careers. You can learn from these common mistakes to avoid making the same ones in the future and to manage your response or reaction when (never if) you make mistakes.

- Note to My 25-Year-Old Self, a candid reflection by top healthcare executives. Each note is a mix of advice from the leader to himself or herself at a young age, general words of wisdom to early careerists, and reminiscences of past experiences and lessons. These leaders are so generous to share their thoughts (even their regrets and mistakes) with us, and we are very thankful.

At the end of some chapters, you will find Additional Resources and References, which we encourage you to check out for more information. At the end of the book, we offer our lists of books that were influential to our professional development and that remain our favorites. And, new to this second edition, we include a Frequently Asked Questions (and Answers) section, sharing a handful of the most frequent queries we receive from our mentees and readers, and our answers to them.

One more thing: We understand the temptation to skim and skip chapters, but please don't! Here's why: We arranged the sequence of the chapters so that one lays the foundation for the next, which in turn builds on the ideas of the previous one and sets up another layer for the next. It's an interlocking chain. If you jump ahead, you may miss a detail that links one concept or strategy to another and thus lose the full message. Read this book over breakfast, on the commuter train to work or internship, or when you get tired of scrolling through your social media feed or playing addictive games on your phone. We don't care where you do it or how long it takes you. Just please read it from beginning to end.

CONCLUSION

We consider *The Emerging Healthcare Leader: A Field Guide* the beginning of our conversation with you, not the end. Please reach out to us. We can't wait to hear about your journey.

Laurie Baedke and Natalie Lamberton

PART I

Laying a Solid Foundation for a Successful You

No one has to tell you that healthcare management is complex; we're sure your professors, industry mentors, colleagues and bosses, textbooks and field literature, and personal or professional experiences have fully briefed you on that fact. The parade of challenges in a healthcare organization—including state and federal regulations, medical errors and other quality problems, accreditation mandates, revenue loss and cost-control issues, reimbursement cuts, technology obsolescence and advancements, workforce and patient demands, and physician alignment or engagement—is daunting. It's enough to make even seasoned managers and leaders scratch their heads.

No one has to tell you that this work—the work you have chosen to do—is mentally, physically, and emotionally draining. But it's fulfilling, too, and surprising (in a good way) and fun (in a thrilling, roller-coaster kind of way).

No one has to tell you that the care delivery sector in which you're serving—including hospitals, medical centers, health systems, physician group practices, and other small and big facilities—is a large industry inside a huge industry inside the massive, high-stakes US healthcare system. It's like a turducken submerged in a pressure cooker.

No one has to tell you that the professionals who make up the healthcare delivery workforce—from the primary care physicians and specialists to the nurses to the advanced practice clinicians to the administrators and senior leaders—are highly skilled, well educated and trained, credentialed, licensed, certified, and/or registered.

You know all this already. What you may not know is how you—the recent addition to the field—can stand out and start making your mark amid the constant swirl of changes and crises in your organization. This is where part I of this book comes in.

Part I consists of chapters that discuss the fundamental principles, approaches, behaviors, and perspectives that you need to understand and then apply so that you can thrive in the healthcare workplace—or any workplace, for that matter. We stuffed these chapters with practical strategies, examples, mini-stories, recommendations, and glimpses into our own experiences. We did that to make the concepts as clear, relatable, and applicable as possible.

Remember this: The first decade of your career is your proving ground. Do as much as possible with that time and the opportunities that come your way, and do it while conducting yourself as well as you can. Part I shows you how to do that.

Note to My 25-Year-Old Self

When I was 25, I transitioned from being the head nurse for a medical/surgical unit and an intensive care unit to being the director of professional relations for a different hospital in another state. That was good, because one piece of advice I followed—and one I would give others—is don't ever take the same job twice. When my husband and I were being transferred to new jobs, I was offered another head nurse position. I turned it down. It was a bigger hospital and a different patient population, but the job would not have given me the opportunity to learn anything new.

One of the things I wish I had known then was this: Know your strengths and weaknesses, and find positions that build on your strengths and minimize your weaknesses. At 25, I assumed I was (or at least could become) good at almost anything. I didn't appreciate what I have come to understand over the years: Everyone has natural talents. That doesn't mean you can't learn other skills, but certain abilities are more ingrained in your personality than others. As an example, I excel at strategic thinking. That is a good thing in that it allows me to be a creative and innovative leader, but it is a bad thing in the face of financial restraints. Therefore, I know now that I must surround myself with folks who have their feet planted firmly in financial reality and can bring me back down to earth when needed.

Another thing I wish I had appreciated at age 25 was this: To be comfortable in your career, you must understand and accept your personal values and know the limits to which you will push them. When I was 25, I thought I needed to accept whatever my boss told me to do or to believe. As I have grown, I understand that not every boss in the world has a value system that is compatible with my personal values. When I look back on my career, I realize that the times I was most dissatisfied or uncomfortable with my work life had something to do with the variation between what I personally believed was right and what my boss or the organization I worked for believed. If your value system is not in sync with that of a potential employer, run—don't walk—away.

Finally, there is something I instinctively knew at 25 that I would tell any 25-year-old today. I am asked many times, "How did you get where you are today?" My answer is this: I volunteered for it. That doesn't mean I raised my hand and said, "OK, I'll be the CEO!" It means I have given every employer more than what they paid me for. If I see a job that needs to be done, I volunteer to do it—whether or not it is in my job description. I believe that is one of the reasons I came to the attention of those in the position to hire me and advance my career. More important, volunteering has always given me a feeling of ownership and satisfaction in the organizations for which I have worked. It is part of the reason I can wake up every morning and say, "Thank God I get to go to work today." My prayer is that you can do the same.

Signed,
Di Smalley, FACHE
Chairman (2013–2014), American College of Healthcare Executives
Regional President, Mercy/Oklahoma

CHAPTER 1

Learn Self-Awareness

And you? When will you begin that long journey into yourself?

—Rumi, thirteenth-century Persian poet

Reading Points

- What Is Self-Awareness?
- How Can You Gain Self-Awareness?
- What Can Self-Awareness Do for You?

PERSONAL—AND, BY extension, professional—development begins with an introspective self-evaluation. The more honest you are with yourself, the more eager you are to correct your faults or to accentuate your good qualities. This self-scrutiny is one of the hardest things to do for most people, yet it is the most important path to self-awareness. A person who is self-aware, in turn, strives to be authentic, confident but humble, curious and open-minded, and eager to learn and improve. Wouldn't you like to work with or for a person like that? More important, wouldn't you like to be that kind of person?

This chapter discusses what self-awareness means for someone like you—a recent entrant to the healthcare workforce. Here, we define self-awareness, offer common strategies for becoming self-aware, and list just a fraction of its many rewards. We also present examples from our own experiences.

WHAT IS SELF-AWARENESS?

The *Merriam-Webster Dictionary* defines the term as the "knowledge and awareness of your own personality and character" (Merriam-Webster 2017). For the purpose of career growth, let's expand that meaning to include work strengths and weaknesses—related to skills and talents, interpersonal or communication styles, behaviors, habits, and so on. In other words, self-awareness refers to a person's understanding of his or her personal and professional traits, tendencies, behaviors, mind-set, abilities, and limitations.

Admittedly, getting to know yourself may feel unnatural. The self-reflection process is odd, frustrating, and even embarrassing; plus, the deliberate focus on yourself may make you feel like a narcissist. After all, it requires you to lower your defenses and raise your candor. If you've ever had a confrontation in which someone—typically, an authority figure—rattled off what's bad and good about you, then you already have an idea of the discomfort this exercise can cause. The good news is that you do this alone (for the most part), but the better news is that the results of your efforts are noticed and even applauded by those around you.

Being self-aware can yield many positives, including

- intimate knowledge of your character, strengths and weaknesses, and interpersonal style;
- better interactions and relationships, because you understand the need to improve the attitudes and behaviors you have that turn people off;

- greater influence on those around you, because your honesty, humility, and authenticity make you instantly relatable—even trustworthy;
- clearer vision of your career path, because you know what you can, cannot, and must do to advance your career; and
- stronger commitment to lifelong learning and growth, because you acknowledge you're a work in progress and need to continually improve.

All of these benefits may position you for faster career advancement. Note, though, that self-awareness alone is not enough to catapult you into the C-suite. Undoubtedly, you still need the education, knowledge, skills, and abilities to fill those roles and the years of experience and expertise to be truly effective. Self-awareness, however, is an essential foundation—no matter what your short-term and long-term goals are. Why? Put simply, the more you know yourself, the better you can fix what is not working and boost what is working.

Strengths and Weaknesses

The sooner in your career you recognize your strengths, the sooner you can enhance, share, and capitalize on them. And the sooner you acknowledge your weaknesses, the sooner you can improve them; work around them; or minimize their effects on others, your performance, or your reputation. Weaknesses aren't all bad, and they're not all major. But they always have the potential to trip you up or to diminish the value of your strengths.

Suppose a hospital's hiring manager is picking the new director of a patient advocacy office and is considering either Applicant A (master's degree, intern for an award-winning medical center, team player, comes off as cold and a know-it-all) or Applicant B (pursuing a master's degree, fellow in a national association for patient advocates, organized and innovative, painfully shy). The manager will hire the applicant most likely to fulfill the job description and fit the organization's or department's culture. The manager is not going to explain to the one not picked why he or she didn't get the job, leaving the applicant bewildered about what went wrong during the interview, how the resume could be revised, which qualification doesn't match, or what skill set or training is missing. But if the applicant is self-aware (i.e., knows his or her strengths and weaknesses), the result may not be as mysterious. A self-aware applicant may have worked around the weaknesses before this point to ensure they do not upstage the strengths. (Back to the example: Who do you think got the job—Applicant A or Applicant B—and why?)

Although we are proponents of authenticity, or letting your true self shine despite your flaws, we don't condone weaknesses that are or that lead to criminal, unethical, hostile, and harmful acts. Such a mind-set, feelings, and behaviors (e.g., racism, bigotry of any kind, extreme views, verbal and physical abusiveness, harassment of any kind, violent tendencies) have no place anywhere—especially not in healthcare, where people come to help and be helped. These negative traits must not be overlooked or viewed as personality quirks, and they must be addressed immediately.

The goal of identifying your strengths and weaknesses is *not* to transform you into a perfect specimen. (News flash: Nobody is perfect—regardless of how impressive and amazing an individual is; plus, self-aware individuals seek constant learning and improvement, not perfection.) The goal is to know and then to *act* on that information; it's like managing what can be measured, which is a quintessential leadership principle. After all, simply knowing something is useless if nothing comes of it. Take us, for example; we both continue to take stock or self-evaluate, and we do something about our respective discoveries.

Natalie's strengths (or the sweet spots, as we like to refer to them) are innovative thinking, big-picture and detail-oriented focus, persistence or tenacity, inclusive interaction with all the stakeholders in her organization, strategic planning, and crafting and implementing an organizational vision. Her weaknesses include her cheerful personality, which those around her may find off-putting, especially when she's leading staff through tough challenges. In fact, a former board member once asked her, "How are you going to be a leader? You're so small and so happy." Aware that this bubbly disposition could be viewed as an unbecoming trait for a leader, Natalie has worked on moderating the way she comes across. (See chapter 2 to learn how she does it.) And she continues to work on this every day.

On the other hand, Laurie's sweet spot is catalyzing and communicating new businesses, strategies, and change initiatives. She is effective at teaching, coaching, and engaging stakeholders to enable successful execution. She is a strong visionary, just like Natalie. Her weakness is impatience. Because she is task oriented, she focuses on completing one step after another and occasionally forgets (unintentionally) to pause to first align resources and gain support for a new project. Now that she recognizes this tendency, she has made deliberate adjustments.

If you mitigate your weaknesses and leverage your strengths, you are in essence self-managing (the topic of chapter 2). That is, you are taking action based on information you've gathered. More specifically, you are taking charge of your own circumstances and thus the opportunities that come your way. As a result, you can move your career forward—in whatever industry and in whatever direction. And you can do all this efficiently and productively. Score!

Self-Management Example

For many people, the need for self-assessment or self-evaluation does not become obvious until they experience an event or a series of events (the aha moment, the light bulb turning on, the catalyst) that makes them wonder if they should make a change. Such events include a termination, a demotion, a bad performance review, dissatisfaction on the job, or a threat of being downsized. The following example illustrates this scenario and the beginning of self-management.

After graduating with a bachelor's degree in computer science, Jill landed a job with a healthcare software company. She was hired for a position in the customer support department, helping clients customize their software and troubleshooting their problems. She loved math and science in school and assumed that the logical thinking and problem solving required by the job fit her interests and degree well. (Plus, in a tight job market, she considered herself lucky for finding full-time employment—let alone a job that had something to do with her major.) For two years, she struggled to enjoy or find satisfaction with work. She didn't like the repetitive nature of the job or the rigid standards her department had to follow. She craved more, but she didn't know exactly what that meant.

When a position opened in the development side of the company, Jill followed her gut and applied for it. She got the job! She was now responsible for designing software features and enhancements, and she was part of a team that developed programs from the ground up. For the first time, she felt like she was a contributor to the organization's vision and strategic goals, not just a cog in the wheel. Her performance reviews reflected her newfound happiness, and her clients and coworkers constantly complimented her ideas and work.

That's when Jill started thinking about her career—specifically, moving up the organizational ladder; going back to school to obtain certifications, get more training, and update her skills; and joining a national association for healthcare information technology professionals to learn more about the industry. She also began to acknowledge that although she was good at logical thinking and problem solving, she was great at strategic and creative thinking (though she uses both sets of skills in her designs). Soon, she began winning awards and boosting her positive reputation.

Today, Jill looks back at those early years and is thankful for the experience. But she is convinced that if she had taken the time to do more self-reflection earlier (even before she graduated) and then begun self-management—rather than just hanging in there and hoping for things to improve—she could have advanced in the company much sooner.

HOW CAN YOU GAIN SELF-AWARENESS?

There's more than one way to become self-aware. For example, Anthony K. Tjan (2012), founder of a venture capital firm and a contributor to the *Harvard Business Review*, proposes a three-pronged approach: (1) testing and knowing yourself, (2) watching yourself and learning in the process, and (3) understanding others' self-awareness. Plus, many hospitals, health systems, health administration programs at colleges and universities, medical schools, healthcare professional associations, healthcare consultants, physician and executive coaches, and other groups offer seminars and webinars, academic courses, continuing education training, publications (e.g., books, articles, white papers, studies), and other resources on recognizing, honing, and applying self-awareness. Also available are a plethora of personality tests and 360-degree assessments (e.g., Myers-Briggs Type Indicator, Kiersey Temperament Sorter, StrengthsFinder, DiSC, Predictive Index) you can self-administer or pay someone to administer to you.

Our recommendations for gaining self-awareness—or embarking on that journey, because you could spend a lifetime discovering yourself or new things about you—are rooted in the same principles discussed in the existing literature or taught in educational programs. But ours are less formal and start at the ground level—where you are now, instead of where you want to be in the future. The following sections detail steps you can take today.

Embrace Humility

A trademark of self-aware people is humility. Modest people—those who don't brag about their talents and accomplishments but are quick to congratulate or compliment others on theirs—are inspirational. They do everything with integrity and are focused on serving others. They understand, and acknowledge, their weaknesses and constantly invite others to help them improve and grow. They consider their strengths as gifts of luck and opportunity and as products of other people's hard work and generosity. They have a lot to teach (and they do so often), but they insist they are merely students. They are confident in their abilities, but they admit they don't know everything. They treat everyone with respect and recognize their value—regardless of what those people can do, contribute, or help with; they don't use people to advance their own agenda.

Being humble draws people in and thus expands one's sphere of influence. But we admit true humility (not false modesty) takes a lot of discipline and years to cultivate. It may not be easy for young careerists to balance the professional need to make their mark (e.g., showing what you can do, proving your proficiency or expertise, expecting and wanting credit for your contributions, getting seen and heard to land opportunities) with the personal desire to be modest—at least not when they just begin a job. However, it is possible to be a humble young professional. The first step is to get real with yourself.

Commit to Getting Real with Yourself

Just as you need to take basic math before you can take advanced math, you need to adopt basic honesty before you can move on to self-awareness. Without basic honesty, you may find it not only difficult but impossible to admit that you have flaws and limitations, that you need to step outside yourself to gain perspective, that you need help, that you don't know nearly as much as you believe, and that you need to make adjustments.

You can't be honest if you're too proud or not humble. Your pride—which may stem from your achievements, high self-esteem or sense of worth, or upbringing—can block you from seeing the truth. For example, if at a young age you won a prestigious, merit-based award (a scholarship, publication, first place in a competition, or any coveted selection by a distinguished jury), you may view it as proof that you have reached the level of the best and as unwritten permission to feel self-satisfied. By all means, be proud of what you've achieved, but have some perspective, too. An award gives its recipients a start—a chance to do more with their skills, talents, and potential. It shouldn't be used as a pass to boast endlessly, which alienates people. Don't ever think you can learn little else going forward.

Moderate your pride by seeking feedback from those who know you and can be completely honest with you. Feedback is the surest way to gauge the attitudes, perspectives, traits, and behaviors you display to others but don't observe yourself. When you receive feedback, try not to be defensive, because that will only hinder the process. Instead, take notes and ask for clarification if needed. Carefully think about the comments, especially the negative ones, because they are usually the toughest to deliver but the most enlightening. Then, decide how you will act on the information you have.

Doing nothing in response to feedback is a waste of everyone's time and effort. But half-heartedly reacting to feedback is worse, because you may give up the first time you encounter a slight difficulty and then go back to your old behaviors. Taming your pride requires you to go all in, to "lean in" and take the pain and discomfort associated with honest self-reflection.

Develop a Habit of Self-Evaluation

Your behavior, attitude, perspective, motivation, wants, needs, priorities, and preferences evolve as you experience life and career changes. For example, as an unmarried, childless, just-graduated individual, your focus is likely on landing a decent-paying, full-time job in your field of interest. As you learn more skills and gain greater proficiency, your focus may shift to career advancement—a promotion, a lateral move, a job transfer, more training, or a return to school. As your life and career progress to include more obligations and responsibilities (a growing family, a mortgage, or a demanding position that requires community leadership), your focus will shift again. Through all these seasons or stages of life, your strengths and weaknesses and your general mind-set change, too. So you should perform a self-evaluation regularly (e.g., quarterly, annually, after a big project) to ensure that what you know about yourself (self-awareness) is keeping pace with how you've evolved as a person and as a professional.

Regular self-assessment doesn't have to be complicated; the old-school system of jotting down a list of your strengths and weaknesses works well. Review the list immediately; don't procrastinate. Add notes on how you plan to improve, address, or discuss the items that need the most attention. You may set a date of completion for the specific items or leave them open-ended. Whatever you do, make sure you keep this list in mind as you go about your days. Revisit it often, tape it to your desk, enter it into your smartphone, write about it in a private blog or diary, and update it if needed. Again, whatever you do, don't forget it—especially when you get busy.

Here are some questions to guide you while you do a self-assessment:

- Whom do you communicate best with—in your personal life and at work? Why?
- What parts of the job come easiest to you? Hardest?

- What pitfalls seem to sink you every time? What barriers do you have to leap over? Why? How can you avoid them?
- How do you feel when you complete a task or project, especially a challenging one?
- How do your family members, friends, work colleagues, superiors, and others (e.g., CEO, other senior leaders, volunteers, support staff, clinicians, vendors) perceive or describe you? What do you think they say about you behind your back?
- What parts of your job are most gratifying or rewarding?
- What tasks or projects do you tend to dread, avoid, or procrastinate on?
- Do you ask others for feedback after you complete a project or in general?
- Do you think you are making a difference? For whom? For what? How?
- Where in the organization or your personal life are you making the greatest impact?
- Are you growing in your position? If not, why?
- Have you made a mistake or failed at a task? Dissect the circumstances to examine how you can learn from that event.

Regular self-reflection is important, not just for early careerists but also for every professional regardless of industry or job title. People who don't reflect are less self-aware and thus tend to have an interpersonal style that alienates, belittles, and lowers the morale of others. Unchecked, this behavior can negatively affect your performance and efficacy as a leader.

Nurture Your Curiosity

Albert Einstein said, "The important thing is not to stop questioning. Curiosity has its own reason for existing." For our purposes, the reason may be that the US healthcare system needs curious leaders because curious people are fundamentally brave. They are not afraid to pose 101 questions—even the stupid and already answered ones. They are not intimidated to try new things, meet new people, or even retry old things with old people. They don't blink or break a sweat in the face of progress, changes, and challenges. Plus, curious people have a scientific mind; they approach everything with the scientific method—they consider a question or problem, research that question fully, form a hypothesis, test that hypothesis several times, analyze the results of those tests, build a conclusion, and tell everyone about it so that actions can be taken.

Curiosity is a natural impetus for self-awareness. That is, if you are curious, you are eager to find out what and who make you tick—and then you can leverage that discovery to grow personally and professionally and improve performance. And you do all this in a rigorous manner, as a scientist does. If curiosity is one of your strengths, you can perpetuate the learning that brings about and accelerates growth. Plus, the more you learn, the more curious you get.

So how can you nurture that curiosity, that insatiable spirit in you? Ask questions and contemplate the answers. Communicate (either verbally or in writing) with people who interest you and who have unique experiences and opinions. Ask for advice and follow it. It doesn't matter if the advice works; what matters is that you were open to trying it. Read as much as possible, attend lectures or seminars, keep a journal, do a web search and follow relevant links (often you'll end up in a much different place than where you started), and join discussions—but listen much more than talk.

We are all curious in varying degrees and typically about something or someone outside of ourselves. If you turn that curiosity inward, just imagine the kinds of conclusions you could draw about yourself.

WHAT CAN SELF-AWARENESS DO FOR YOU?

As we mentioned, self-awareness offers numerous advantages. The following sections discuss just a few of the many.

Authenticity and Trust

One of the most important benefits of self-awareness is finding the authentic, multidimensional you—the good, the bad, and the ugly of your character. Your authenticity lowers people's defense mechanisms because it tells them, "I'm a work in progress, and I'm trying my best." Authenticity encourages people to level with you, to be kinder, and to accept both the qualities that make you different from them and those that you share.

When you are authentic,

- you don't have a split personality—you speak and act the same way in public (in front of mixed company) as you do in private (in front of only those you trust);
- you make mistakes and poor decisions, but you acknowledge and apologize when you are wrong and you don't blame everyone else;
- you are honest with yourself and those around you, even if your honesty could put you in an unflattering light;
- you can admit "I don't know" and "I need help" without shame;
- you are not afraid to show emotions that may be perceived as weakness, such as sadness, anger (i.e., irritation and exasperation, *not* temper tantrums, abusive conduct, or blind rage), disappointment, fear, confusion, or doubt;
- you express genuine concern for and desire to help with people's predicaments; and

- you practice what you preach and do so according to your own belief system—not according to popular opinion or trendy practice.

This kind of behavior enables you to connect with others and earn their trust.

Stephen M. R. Covey (2008)—son of the late management expert Stephen R. Covey, author of *7 Habits of Highly Effective People*—wrote about instant trust in his book, *The Speed of Trust*. (Instant trust is a relatively new idea that contrasts with the old—but still valid—model of earning trust only after a long time of proving yourself.) The book's subtitle summarizes Covey's thesis about trust: *The One Thing That Changes Everything*. Trust is a currency, and if you have it you can do just about anything. If you are self-aware, you will likely use that currency for good and be transparent about what you do with it.

Influence and Style

Healthcare administration is a stressful 24-7 job, so you need to surround yourself with people whose support you can count on. In addition to the strength of your character (integrity, accountability, credibility), your interpersonal style—whether you're introverted, charismatic, strategic, creative, compassionate, driven, laid back, or something in between—plays a big role in expanding or diminishing your influence over others.

Influence isn't about being liked or being popular; a leader does not worry about who likes him or her. (Generally, when you're kind, you don't have to wonder if people like you. The reverse is also true.) Influence is about understanding your interpersonal style's effect on others and adjusting your approach to forge connections and relationships with those you can help and who will, in turn, help you get things done.

Every interaction you have is both an opportunity for others to judge your personality and character and an opportunity for you to evaluate whether you're conveying your strengths or highlighting your weaknesses. If the former, your influence may grow; if the latter, your influence may suffer.

Ask yourself the following questions when evaluating your style and thus your influence. (Always elaborate on your answers to better explore your thinking or rationale.)

- Am I able to connect with leaders, both the formal and the informal? How?
- Am I able to engage colleagues, staff, bosses, executives, patients, clinicians, and other stakeholders? How?
- Am I drawn to people or processes? Why?
- Am I more comfortable with one-on-one or group interaction? Why?
- Do I tend to say, "let's do it," "you do it," or "I'll do it"?
- How would I and others characterize my style? Am I comfortable with that?
- Do I prefer to deal with the big picture or the details?
- Is planning or implementation my sweet spot?

Confidence

As you become more self-aware, your confidence grows and your anxiety diminishes. The confidence comes from knowing your strengths and weaknesses. When you reach this level of self-awareness, you will no longer be content to sit (and doodle—yep, we know what you're doing) in meetings, half-heartedly listening to the bigwigs discuss the issues and nervously waiting for your turn to report on your project. You will speak up when appropriate, politely but decisively. Beyond meetings, you will get involved in the daily life of the department, unit, or office. You will contribute according to your knowledge and capabilities. You will start acting like a self-aware leader, building relationships, giving compliments and credit to deserving individuals and groups, learning about everything, gaining trust, and managing your career.

One last note: Do not confuse confidence with boastfulness. Boastful people are typically insecure. They have a constant desire to be noticed and praised, and they get validation from people's reactions (especially envy) to their accomplishments. Confident people, on the other hand, are typically secure. They are fully aware of who they are, what they have, what they know, and what they can do. Although they are proud of their accomplishments (and will boast about them only to thank the people who have helped them), they don't gloat or show off. They understand that the true reward comes not from fleeting or even insincere praise but from the tangible outcomes.

Rookie Mistakes

Getting Caught in the Comparison Trap

When was the last time you chided yourself for not having someone else's body or brains or talent or relationship or family? How about that person's car or house or income? How about his or her job title, education, social status, or accomplishments?

It's natural to compare yourself to others. We all do it in one way or another. For example, when Laurie first joined the entrepreneurial (read: independent contracting) world of healthcare consulting, she occasionally thought those with traditional jobs had it better. They received a predictable paycheck every month or every other week, and they didn't

→

have to worry about where their next project would come from. Likewise, other career rookies may long for the salary and benefits their contemporaries earn, may disparage others' professional wins because of jealousy or rivalry, or may become downright depressed and resentful about the opportunities that stubbornly evade them but seem to flow straight to others. Comparisons may be common, but they can trap you in an unproductive, exhausting cycle of coveting, envy, and self-loathing.

To break this cycle, focus on what you have contributed and what you have achieved using your own wit, skills, and courage. Then, figure out what you need to do to be happy with the choices you made. That's exactly what Laurie did. She accepted that it's not greener on the other side and took an inventory of her life and career. She realized her job allowed her the time, space, and flexibility that traditional jobs lacked. She could build lasting and rewarding relationships, engage in a variety of challenging work, pursue leadership opportunities in professional associations, and entertain limitless opportunities—both in and out of work.

Pretending to Be Someone You're Not

An extreme consequence of comparing yourself to others is subconsciously or consciously absorbing their desirable qualities into your own persona. For example, if you admire your Facebook friend's volunteer activities, you might add that information to your resume or mention it during a job interview even if you haven't volunteered anywhere before. The same goes for work experiences, schools attended, hobbies, social and political affiliations, honors received, papers published, and even personal philosophies. You might think that doing so is harmless, the detail will impress other

→

people, and your little white lie will not get discovered. But you are wrong.

First, you are committing a form of identity theft (at worst) and an unequivocal, untenable lie (at the least). Second, the good impression you might leave on a job screener is fleeting when compared with the long-lasting bad impression you will leave on everyone else. Third, hiring managers and human resources staff often verify resume details and the claims you make during an interview; at the very least, they will check your online profiles. Fourth, even if you get away with this unseemly tactic, the job (or the people you lied to) will eventually force you to apply what you claimed to know or have done. If you can't back up your words with action, you can't expect to remain in that position.

To avoid that drama, just be authentic. Own who you are, and don't dare apologize for it. Remember that the online and offline personae most people display in public are the edited versions and not the rough drafts. In reality, their lives are less impressive. Fibbing only causes you stress and confusion about your career direction.

Being a Watcher, Not a Doer

When you're just starting your career, it's sometimes easiest to adopt the herd mentality and go along with the crowd. For example, in a meeting everyone agrees with the boss that option A is the best resolution for problem B. You nod your head and smile along with the group, even if your instinct tells you there's a better solution.

That's understandable. The healthcare workplace is very intimidating. Decisions made there are often either

→

life-or-death or affect a large cluster of people. Everything is a process with multiple steps. People walk and talk fast, and you're expected to keep up. Early in your career, almost everyone is older and more experienced than you. Thus, your natural response is to anxiously listen and observe, not participate.

However, you were hired for a reason, so show everyone what you can do. Listen intently but join the conversation as well. State your opinions and back them up with evidence, which means you have to do your homework and prepare as much as possible. Volunteer for projects that will showcase your skills, but also be willing to take risks and challenges. Take advantage of as many opportunities as you can to learn and contribute with gusto. Your enthusiasm, eagerness, and confidence will be duly noted.

Investing Too Much in Your Weaknesses, Not Enough in Your Strengths

Don't get us wrong; we recommend improvement in all areas, and minimizing or eliminating weaknesses is a beneficial exercise. However, you should not pour all of your precious resources—time, money, physical and mental energy, and patience—into correcting a personality or professional deficiency while ignoring your promising qualities and innate talents. Strengths need as much (or even more) attention as weaknesses, depending on the position you hold.

Suppose you are terrible at small talk but excellent at public or group speaking. Determine which skill is more useful to the job you have today and the job you want in the near future. Then, devote an appropriate amount of resources to developing each skill. Ask yourself what you'll get out of

→

each investment. For example, would learning how to chat improve your interactions, make your daily duties easier, or increase the chances of landing your dream job? Likewise, would refining your public speaking make you more persuasive and informative, boost your department's/organization's reputation both internally and in the community, help get you a raise or promotion, or give you a competitive edge?

Visualize weighing on a scale the resources you put in against the results you get out. If the resources are much heavier than the results, then you can lighten the resources load significantly. This scale should not balance; the results should be heavier than the resources. More bang for your buck!

Unfortunately, many new careerists (including us when we were starting out) favor fixing weaknesses over enhancing strengths. Many human resources departments and supervisors do as well. But we all need to change that mind-set so that we're not wasting our resources on things that may not pay off in the long run.

Remember These

- Self-awareness refers to a person's understanding of his or her personal and professional traits, tendencies, abilities, and limitations.
- A person who is self-aware strives to be authentic, confident but humble, curious and open-minded, and eager to learn and improve.
- If you mitigate weaknesses and leverage strengths, you are self-managing or taking charge of your own circumstances and thus the opportunities that come your way.

$\rightarrow$

- Do a regular self-assessment to ensure your self-awareness is keeping pace with your personal and professional evolution.

- Regular self-reflection is important not just for early careerists but also for every professional regardless of industry or job title. People who don't reflect are less self-aware and thus tend to have an interpersonal style that alienates, belittles, and lowers the morale of others.

- The trademark of self-aware people is humility.

- You can't be honest if you're not humble or if you're too proud. Your pride can block you from seeing the truth.

- Curiosity is a natural impetus for self-awareness. If you are curious, you are eager to find out what makes you tick—and then you can leverage that discovery to grow personally and professionally and improve performance.

- One of the most important benefits of self-awareness is finding the authentic, multidimensional you—the good, the bad, and the ugly. Your authenticity lowers people's defense mechanisms, which leads them to connect with and trust you.

- As you become more self-aware, your confidence grows and your anxiety diminishes.

- Do not confuse confidence with boastfulness. Boastful people are typically insecure, while confident people are typically secure.

REFERENCES

Covey, S. M. R. 2008. *The Speed of Trust: The One Thing That Changes Everything.* New York: Free Press.

Merriam-Webster. 2017. "Self-Awareness." Accessed November 30. www.merriam-webster.com/dictionary/self-awareness.

Tjan, A. K. 2012. "How Leaders Become Self-Aware." *Harvard Business Review* Blog Network. Posted July 19. http://blogs.hbr.org/2012/07/how-leaders-become-self-aware.

ADDITIONAL RESOURCES

Green Peak Partners. 2014. "When It Comes to Business Leadership, Nice Guys Finish First." http://greenpeakpartners.com/uploads/Green-Peak_Cornell-University-Study_What-predicts-success.pdf.

Tobak, S. 2013. "Seven Signs You're Not as Self-Aware as You Think." www.inc.com/steve-tobak/7-signs-youre-not-as-self-aware-as-you-think.html.

CHAPTER 2

Practice Self-Management

We cannot change what we are not aware of, and once we
are aware, we cannot help but change.

—Sheryl Sandberg, chief operating officer, Facebook

Reading Points

- How Self-Management Works

- Why Personality Matters

- When Weaving Work and Life Is Better Than Balancing
  Them

- What Would a Lifelong Learner Do?

NOW THAT YOU'VE done some self-reflection and have gotten
acquainted with your strengths and weaknesses, you may wonder
what's next. Self-management—that's what.

Essentially, self-management is about being accountable for
your actions—in general or for a specific purpose—while relying
on your strengths and resources. When you manage yourself, you
are policing your own behavior and adjusting it to attain a desired
outcome. This requires not only self-awareness but also mental

toughness and discipline, because self-management could lead you through ugly and awkward choices and eventually to change.

Have you ever been on a strict diet? Ever had to live on a small budget? Ever had to position yourself for a raise or a promotion? Answering yes to any of these questions means you have done a form of self-management. This chapter discusses how self-management works and what personal and professional areas in your life can be enhanced by it.

HOW SELF-MANAGEMENT WORKS

Self-management is mind-bogglingly useful. Many individuals, groups, and industries apply self-management to many types of goals and objectives. Want to reduce stress, save money for retirement, monitor an illness, or meet and mingle with the right people? Then self-management is just the thing for you! We know this sounds like a too-good-to-be-true course taught at your local community center, but the process is legit (i.e., legitimately helpful and legitimately awesome).

The components common in self-management include the following:

1. Identifying the problem to be solved, the goal to be accomplished, or the task to be performed (What do I want to do?)
2. Selecting the method, timeline, and strategies to be followed (How do I want to do it, and when?)
3. Monitoring your progress along the way, and making adjustments or corrections as necessary (How am I doing?)
4. Analyzing the outcome (How did I do? What did I learn?)

Of course, the components change according to who is self-managing and for what purpose and industry. Of course, no one is required to follow these components (after all, they're not steps), but some people use them as a guideline to organize their self-management effort.

These components clearly convey that self-management involves choices, and those choices are influenced by self-awareness. For example, if you've discovered that aversion to change is a weakness, you could opt to improve it or live with it. If you pick improvement, you are faced with myriad strategies for accepting and dealing with change. If you choose to live with it, you must consider the consequences. Among these consequences is the possibility that you will experience slower career growth than your peers despite your superior strengths. As we mentioned in chapter 1, some weaknesses eclipse strengths; aversion to change is an unfortunate weakness to have in an industry that is known for its constant changes.

Now a warning: Practicing self-management doesn't automatically lead to great outcomes. You could set goals, choose the best strategies, and check your progress periodically all you want. But if you're not doing the work necessary to change or adjust the behavior, you won't see any improvement.

WHY PERSONALITY MATTERS

Your personality—the character traits that make you *you*—is one of the many factors that make people want to engage with or disengage from you. That personality comes across in your interactions, whether personal or professional. So managing your interpersonal style and how you are perceived is important. (See chapter 4 for a complete discussion of character.)

By managing, we don't mean that you should pretend to be someone other than your true self or conceal (but not reverse) your bad qualities. We mean that you should continually assess the impression you leave (good or bad) after an interaction and then amend the behavior that diminishes your message and intention.

For example, for Natalie, self-management is about paying attention to people's reactions to her. She asks for and accepts others' feedback and adds that to the information she gathers on her own so that she can process all of it internally. She's aware of her bubbly, perky, or exuberant disposition, the inner joy that shows on her face; she's always smiling. On the surface, this is awesome because she is approachable. Plus, imagine an executive who is upbeat even at the crack of dawn! But this trait isn't everyone's cup of tea. It could undermine her professional edge, not to mention the gravity of her position. It might lead those who don't know Natalie to dismiss her as silly and thus not to be taken seriously, but that's the farthest from the truth. Since she discovered this fact, she has taken action. In face-to-face interactions, Natalie deliberately controls her tone of voice, hand and body movements, and facial expressions. This way, her disposition does not distract from or get in the way of the message she's trying to convey. In stressful situations, Natalie does the same thing. She remains even-keeled and doesn't jump to conclusions or plot the next course of action before all the facts are known. She listens to explanations and takes a few minutes before responding.

For Laurie, the focus of self-management is on reining in her intensity. Although she embraces it and deems it an asset (as it has enabled her to achieve much success in both the entrepreneurial and corporate worlds and has motivated others to do the same), she also recognizes that her intensity can be overwhelming for her coworkers. She considers feedback as her "breakfast of champions" and constantly seeks it from peers and others in her community. Talking through circumstances in which she needs help allows her to adjust her interpersonal style and perform at the highest level possible.

Remember, there's no wrong type of personality—all types are valid and valuable. Continually managing that personality is key to improving your interpersonal style, expanding your influence, and cultivating your leadership style.

WHEN WEAVING WORK AND LIFE IS BETTER THAN BALANCING THEM

When we were just starting our careers, one of the biggest work-place trends was work–life balance, the idea that employees (especially working mothers) could nurture a career and a family in equal measure. Later, the trend became life–work balance, the notion that employees value time off to spend with their friends and family more than they value money. Today, both concepts still exist, but more people are asking, Is there such a thing as balance?

Balance implies that you are forcing two separate entities to cooperate with each other, to give and to take as necessary. But neither life nor work is a good sharer. One always demands more than the other, and often both demand so much at the same time. If one doesn't relent to the other, you could end up damaging both. That's not a comforting scenario.

A new question has emerged: Why not accept that the two entities are woven together (or integrated) and that one doesn't end when the other begins? This question reflects a self-aware perspective. It recognizes that work and life are not the same, but they are not separate either. After all, who among us has not checked or responded to work e-mail on our day off? And who among us has not made a personal phone call during work hours?

As you manage your work and life activities, keep your priorities straight and make adjustments as you see fit. Don't stress out if some of your activities overlap, because they often will. For example, completing a specific project—like a month-end or year-end strategic plan or budget forecast—may consume a substantial amount of time. This type of project might clash with the timing of a life event, such as the birth of a baby, the death or illness of a loved one, or preparation for a wedding. These life events may cause you to lean more heavily into or away from your work obligations, but eventually things will go back to normal.

Balancing calls for compartmentalizing work and life obligations. If you are trying to balance, you might miss either a work or a personal event because you might think personal time shouldn't encroach on work time, and vice versa. That thought is unrealistic, and it causes an imbalance because you become preoccupied with the task you are not supposed to be doing (e.g., completing a departmental analysis) so you can't focus on the task you are supposed to be doing (e.g., going to the gym). In this age of the Internet, telecommuting, social networking, smartphones, and innovative living and working arrangements, it makes more sense to integrate than to separate the professional and the personal (Schawbel 2014).

Weaving life into work and vice versa is not new; many people have been doing it for years. It's just that we hadn't given it a name yet and maybe we had been doing it all wrong. Having said that, the essential idea of a balanced life is still good. By *balanced*, we mean the personal should be given the same value and respect as the professional (and vice versa), and adjustments should be made to allow for one priority to overtake the other when necessary. The trend toward work–life integration has greater potential for sustainability, both for us as individuals and for the organizations that we serve.

The Personal Cost of Professional Success

James Andrews, MD, is an American orthopedic surgeon renowned for his expert skills, success rate, and significant contributions to the field of sports medicine. He has been a sought-after surgeon for both amateur and professional athletes; among his star patients were Michael Jordan, Drew Brees, and Jack Nicklaus. He helped found the Andrews Institute (where he still practices at age 75) and the American Sports Medicine Institute (which churns out research about sports injuries and treatments). He introduced to his field some of the most innovative surgical and rehabilitation technologies still in use today (Helyar 2007). He has mentored up-and-coming orthopedists, has written a book, and gives motivational speeches.

Andrews makes himself available 24-7; in fact, always being available is one of his trademarks. By all accounts, he is on his cell phone when he's not consulting with patients or in the operating room. He fields calls not only from patients and their families but also from trainers, team owners, other orthopedic surgeons, physical therapists, and coaches (to name a few). And his productivity is legendary: At his peak, he performed 1,200 surgeries in one year, while the average orthopedist does about 400 annually (Eden 2013).

Andrews is likely envied by many. He's smart. He's accomplished. He's loved by those he has helped and continues to help. He's powerful and well connected. He's a one-of-a-kind asset to his field. From outside appearances, he has it all—like so many achievers people aspire to be and measure their accomplishments against. But what these comparisons tend *not* to show are the personal sacrifices made and the price tag attached to achieving a tremendous amount of success. For Andrews, one trade-off was a heart attack in 2006.

When you reflect on your American dream, consider the trade-offs (there will always be some):

- What are you giving up now? What will you be willing to give up later?
- What are you getting in return now? What do you expect to get in return later?
- Is the dream worth pursuing at the expense of everything else?
- When you look back on your life, will you have any regrets? Why or why not?

Your answers to these questions (and others) can guide you in managing your work and life priorities today. In addition, remember to consider the seasons of life. Freedom to invest in both personal and professional pursuits will ebb and flow as you go through those seasons.

WHAT WOULD A LIFELONG LEARNER DO?

Personal and professional development does not have to be expensive, like enrolling in a leadership immersion program or engaging an executive coach (though both are terrific options). It could be small and free but ongoing, like asking for feedback, interviewing an inspirational leader, listening to audiobooks or podcasts during your commute, and staying connected with your network. These and other such investments pay off in a variety of ways. Lifelong learning is not just informative; it also strengthens relationships, offers opportunities for change, enhances interpersonal skills, and reveals lasting lessons.

If you are a lifelong learner, you

- are disciplined (so that you can stick with development throughout your career),
- are curious (so that you never stop asking questions and finding answers), and
- have the right attitude (so that you can always be supportive of and enthusiastic about learning).

A self-aware person with a goal of becoming a lifelong learner would devise and follow a plan for cultivating her discipline, curiosity, and positive attitude. Plus, she would try the methods outlined in the following sections.

Ask for Feedback

We meet many professionals struggling in one or more skill areas. When we recommend that they ask for feedback, they typically look like they've had a light-bulb moment. Although they aren't strangers to the idea of feedback, they've never solicited it and never thought it could help get them out of their bind. But yes, it can. Let us count the ways:

1. *The act of asking for feedback delivers you from the mind-set that you're on your own.* It is your unspoken (and maybe subconscious) acknowledgment that you are surrounded by people who care about your welfare. Plus, people feel honored to be asked for their honest opinions; that endears you to them.

2. *Feedback yields significant objective and subjective information.* Sift through the advice and pick out what could work for your situation. Take the criticisms seriously but not defensively; correct the wrongs and don't attack the messengers. Be grateful for the compliments and remind yourself of them when you feel doubtful about your talents and abilities.

3. *Feedback points you in a direction.* That path may not be clear yet, but feedback eases your worries that you'll be stuck in one place. In other words, feedback gives you information that you can turn into an improvement or a development plan, and it's up to you to follow it.

4. *The feedback process humbles you.* Asking for, receiving, and analyzing feedback—whether you do it in person or electronically—can bruise the ego (especially if the ego belongs to an overly confident person). This is not a bad thing, because it helps you develop a thick skin for the greater, more ego-busting challenges you'll encounter later in your career.

People are almost always willing to help, so give them a chance to do so. Ask for feedback from your mentor, boss, significant other, coworkers, past and current teachers, real-life friends, social media friends, parents, siblings, and anyone you have meaningful contact with on a regular basis. Don't be afraid that they'll say yes; be afraid that they'll say no, because that would mean you'd miss out on a chance to learn.

Interview an Inspirational Leader

You might not have studied journalism, but you don't need to be a reporter to have a question-and-answer session with a leader you admire. This leader doesn't have to be an executive working in a healthcare facility (although do approach these executives); he or she could be the chair of your health administration program, the head of a private quality-improvement organization, a physician or nurse leader, a member or chair of a hospital board, a new colleague you met at the American College of Healthcare Executives (ACHE) Congress on Healthcare Leadership or in your local ACHE chapter, or any other remarkable individuals in your (presumably healthcare) workplace or field.

This interview doesn't have to be formal; it could take place over coffee or lunch, e-mail, or the phone. You could schedule it for one hour once a month, for at least 12 solid hours of learning per year. Be honest with the leaders about your intentions (e.g., you'd like to learn from their experiences, successes, and mistakes and to hear their insights). And assure them that you will not publish, post, or leak notes from your conversation unless you have their permission to do so.

Leaders might decline your request for an interview because they are typically very busy and may not be comfortable sharing details of their life with a stranger. But try anyway. The experience of reaching out to someone inspirational is, on its own, educational.

Stay Connected with Your Network

If you're like many people, you probably do this: (1) attend an industry event (like ACHE's Congress), a seminar, or an alumni reunion; (2) see old friends and colleagues and meet other professionals; (3) exchange business cards and promise to stay in touch;

and (4) forget about the whole thing. No harm done, right? Not exactly.

When you're new to a field, you must put extra effort into maintaining (not just building) a professional network. You shouldn't merely collect business cards and handshakes. You should start conversations and keep them going.

For example, every week, e-mail one colleague in your network, just to check in and get to know the person more. Ask how he or she is doing, give a brief update about your life when appropriate (don't make the e-mail about you), and refer to something you discussed last time as that could still be a concern you could help with. Don't ask for a favor from your contacts each time you reach out; in fact, don't ask for a favor for a long time. Asking for favors is the fastest way to lose them and to develop a reputation for being opportunistic and needy. (Note that these suggestions still apply if you call, text, snail mail, Snap, or Tweet instead of e-mail. Learn your connections' preferred media, and let them know yours.) Once you've established rapport, you might recommend someone in your network your colleague would find value in getting to know. Share an article you've read that might be insightful or relevant to your colleague's work, or congratulate that colleague when you hear of his or her accomplishments. And voilà, you're functioning as a true networker!

Your network is a great source for many things, including feedback and recommendations for leaders you could interview. And so is your mentor, with whom you should retain a connection. To express your appreciation for all the lessons and time your mentor has freely shared with you, write a thank-you note regularly (e.g., several times a year). In addition, you could invite your mentor to join you in educational activities, such as listening to a podcast of interest, attending an industry lecture or seminar, and reading and discussing a book or two. This way, you're not only spending quality time but also learning together.

Go Green, Stay Green

Andrews imparts some great wisdom for physicians and nonphysicians alike. One of our favorites is "If you're green, you're growing—and if you're ripe, you're next to rotten." (He attributes this maxim to his mentor, Jack Hughston, MD.) This saying is meant to remind emerging leaders like you that you are in the right place and that your newness is an asset because it keeps you open for learning, maturing, evolving, and improving. Although you may have just the basic level of knowledge, skills, and abilities necessary (but not yet the instincts and mastery that come from years of practice), you have the desire and hunger to learn. Don't underestimate that.

In contrast, Andrews warns you of the decline that many (but not all) seasoned professionals feel. By *rotten*, he doesn't mean that these people are bad; he means that they have lost their sense of wonder, enthusiasm, and passion for their profession. They are now mechanically carrying out their day-to-day duties to protect the status and income level they've earned. But they have stopped developing themselves, and they likely haven't been self-aware for decades.

In other words, going green is an analogy for stoking that fire inside you for learning and growth. Anyone can go green, no matter their age, job title, or level of experience. Self-aware leaders work hard to stay green and promote the idea to their staffers, protégés, and colleagues.

So, stay green! How? The answers are throughout this book.

Remember These

- When you manage yourself, you are policing your own behavior and adjusting it to attain a desired outcome.
- Many individuals, groups, and industries apply self-management to many types of goals and objectives.

$\rightarrow$

- Self-management involves choices, and those choices are influenced by self-awareness.
- Your personality is one of the many factors that make people want to engage with or disengage from you. That personality comes across in your interactions, so managing how you are perceived is important.
- Your personal life should be given the same value and respect as your professional life (and vice versa), and you should adjust to allow for one priority to overtake the other when necessary.
- Lifelong learning is not just informative; it also strengthens relationships, offers opportunities for change, enhances interpersonal skills, and reveals lasting lessons.
- When you reflect on your own American dream, consider the trade-offs between professional success and personal happiness as well as the seasons in life.

REFERENCES

Eden, S. 2013. "The Doctor Will Save You Now." *ESPN*. Published September 17. http://espn.go.com/espn/story/_/id/9669812/celebrated-orthopedist-james-andrews-treats-robert-griffin-iii-bryce-harper-espn-magazine.

Helyar, J. 2007. "Dr. James Andrews Still Works on the Cutting Edge." *ESPN*. Published September 20. http://sports.espn.go.com/espn/news/story?id=3024046.

Schawbel, D. 2014. "Work Life Integration: The New Norm." *Forbes*. Published January 21. www.forbes.com/sites/danschawbel/2014/01/21/work-life-integration-the-new-norm/.

ADDITIONAL RESOURCE

Chappelow, C. 2012. "Strive for Work–Life Integration, Not Balance." *Fast Company*. Published March 16. www.fastcompany.com/1825042/strive-work-life-integration-not-balance.

Note to My 25-Year-Old Self

As I consider advice that might have helped me early in my career, much comes to mind. It is more than simply telling myself, "You just don't know how much you don't know." Often, people say they wish they knew that when they started. The reality is, you have decent book knowledge, just not much experience. The most valuable input I can share includes learning to listen well, live fearlessly, care for people, protect your home life, and be a person of great integrity.

Listen more . . . listen *way* more! Ask questions about people and their jobs and the implications of their clinical and operational decisions. Ask them why they chose healthcare. Find out what they like and don't like and how you can make things better. Listen to what they say and how they say it. Listen to what is not said. Observe. Probe. Learn.

When looking for work, interview that organization as well. Ask good questions. Listen carefully to the responses. Look for a boss and a culture that reflect your core values and an employer who cares about you and your career. Be prepared for the interview— not just for the questions you think they will ask you but also for the questions you will ask them. Give thought to the kinds of answers you expect and want to hear. It will tell you a lot about the people and culture. Err on the side of formality, not informality.

Live fearlessly! Don't be afraid of taking risks or making mistakes. We learn from mistakes, and you will never accomplish great things without taking risks. If you don't agree with a policy, a program, a direction, or a decision, challenge it. Do it respectfully, at an appropriate time, and in the appropriate place or setting, but do it! Don't accept the status quo just because it is easy or the cultural norm. Don't be afraid to push back. Also, don't be afraid of losing your job. Living and working in fear is counterproductive and unhealthy. If you lose your job because you disagree or challenge the leadership, it probably wasn't the right organization or job anyway. There are always other jobs for bright, talented, energetic, and hardworking young leaders.

People are more important than the tasks they do each day. Take time to get to know the employees and the physicians. Never forget that they are people first; they are moms and dads and husbands and wives and sisters and brothers and friends. They have hobbies and lives outside of work. Without being intrusive, get to know something about them that is not work related. Ask questions; show genuine interest in your team. Again, listen, observe, care.

Go home. The work will always be there tomorrow. Family may not be. Home life needs to be your most important priority, and if things are going well at home, they will usually be good at work. If you are single, it is still important to go home, get away, and leave work behind. Take vacations—real vacations where you don't check e-mail and stay on the phone half the time. Work will go on without you! Really! By the way, this advice applies not only to you but to your people as well. Create an environment where you encourage your team to keep home as their most important priority. There are no winners in the illusion of a contest for who works the longest days or the most hours!

You already know this, but character counts more than anything else. Ask yourself important questions about your own behavior. Are you reliable? Can others count on you to do what you say you will do and when you say you will do it? Are you characterized as one who has a good work ethic and demonstrates honesty in all situations? Do you talk about others behind their back other than to praise them? Finally, make sure there are members of your team who will hold you accountable by telling you what you *need* to hear and not what you *want* to hear.

There is some obvious stuff for leaders that should not go unsaid. Ethical behavior must always come before all else—never sacrifice integrity. Provide service to others without self-interest—service above self. And finally, whatever you do, do it with excellence—always do your best!

Now go serve others, and have a blast! Healthcare is the greatest career. It's not a job, it's not even just a career; to those who lose themselves in it, it's a calling.

Signed,
Donald R. Avery, FACHE
Governor (2008–2011), American College of Healthcare Executives
President and CEO, Fairview Park Hospital

The Emotionally Intelligent Leader: Habits, Practices, and Attributes of Executive Excellence

One can have no smaller or greater mastery than
mastery of oneself.

—*Leonardo da Vinci*

Contrary to the opinion of many people, leaders are not
born. Leaders are made, and they are made by effort and
hard work.

—*Vince Lombardi*

Reading Points

- Beyond "Smart"
- What Is Emotional Intelligence?
- Emotional Intelligence and Leadership
- Emotional Intelligence Matters
- Gender Differences
- Can Emotional Intelligence Be Learned?
- How to Develop Your Emotional Intelligence

HAVE YOU EVER wondered why certain individuals just seem to accelerate in their careers? They weren't necessarily 4.0 GPA students, but when your paths cross now, they seem to have a rocket strapped to their back. These super-successes are being promoted, advancing their careers quickly, leading others, and spearheading new initiatives. What sets them apart from the rest? In this chapter, we explore their secret—the one ingredient that every successful executive possesses and hones through every stage of her or his career.

BEYOND "SMART"

Our industry and organizations nationwide are filled with individuals who "check all the boxes." Their resume—their degrees, certifications, credentials, and work experience (heck, even their home address, subdivision, and country club membership)—fulfills all the requirements of the position they're employed to perform. Developing strategic plans, implementing new processes, writing budgets, analyzing data—executing these tasks makes one a tactician. But true leadership requires collaboration. This next level of leadership also includes navigating change with others and influencing outcomes through others—plus large doses of empathy, social and relational savvy, and self-awareness.

Let's face it—the hardest parts of any job are rarely found in the tactical. Clear-cut problems are easily resolved with more information or training. The greatest challenge of work involves the human quotient.

Emotional intelligence is the variable that separates the tacticians from the true leaders, the smarty-pants from the exceptional executives. The emotionally intelligent leader pursues mastery of both the tactical and the human elements of his or her job. In this chapter, we explore what emotional intelligence is, share research that explains why it's important for success, and lay out a few ways you can continue to develop it as you progress in your career.

WHAT IS EMOTIONAL INTELLIGENCE?

The *Merriam-Webster Dictionary* (2017) defines *intelligence quotient* (IQ) as

> 1: a number used to express the apparent relative intelligence of a person, such as
>
>> a: the ratio of the mental age (as reported on a standardized test) to the chronological age multiplied by 100,
>>
>> b: a score determined by one's performance on a standardized test relative to the average performance of others of the same age.
>
> 2: proficiency in or knowledge of a specified subject. Example: "Nobody questioned his hockey IQ."

By contrast, Daniel Goleman, PhD, an author, psychologist, and science journalist, defines *emotional intelligence* as

> 1: the ability to understand oneself and to empathize with others.
>
> 2: the capacity for recognizing our own feelings and those of others, for motivating ourselves, and for managing emotions well in ourselves and in our relationships.

How does Goleman's definition apply to the emerging, developing leader? Does emotional intelligence even matter in the workplace?

EMOTIONAL INTELLIGENCE AND LEADERSHIP

If you had to list the most common attributes and competencies traditionally associated with leadership, what would they be? Traits such as intelligence, toughness, determination, and vision probably spring to mind.

What about emotionally intelligent people? What would you list as their resounding characteristics? You might picture them with a high level of self-awareness and self-regulation. They are highly motivated and empathetic, and they possess strong social and relationship management skills.

The two lists of traits don't seem to overlap much. So does emotional intelligence even matter when it comes to leadership potential? The short answer: yes. As we will explore in this chapter, many experts argue that emotional intelligence is more—perhaps even much more—important than IQ.

A 2012 article published by *Forbes* magazine proposed that IQ alone is barely an indicator when it comes to predicting success and professional achievement, and that a high IQ does not guarantee you will stand out among the crowd (Jensen 2012).

The management theory called the Peter Principle states that those who are selected for promotions are chosen more for their performance in their current role than for their technical knowledge related to the newly intended role. Could your ability to self-assess, collaborate, empathize, and motivate yourself and influence others really get you promoted above your technical skill level? Let's dig into the research to find out.

Goleman and *Harvard Business Review*

Goleman, who reported for the *New York Times* for 12 years on topics related to the brain and behavioral sciences, first applied the concept of emotional intelligence to the business world when he published the results of his research in *Harvard Business Review* in 1998. His study, conducted at nearly 200 large, global companies, found direct connections between emotional intelligence and business results.

Goleman's objective was to determine which personal capabilities drove outstanding performance in these companies, and to what degree they did so. He measured three main categories:

1. Technical skills, such as accounting, business planning, and project management
2. Cognitive abilities, such as analytical reasoning
3. Competencies demonstrating emotional intelligence, such as the ability to work with others and effectiveness in leading change

As expected, he found that technical skills and cognitive abilities were important drivers of outstanding performance, but considering all three categories as ingredients of success, emotional intelligence was two times more important than the others for job roles at all levels. "Research clearly shows that emotional intelligence is the sine qua non of leadership. Without it, a person can have the best training in the world, an incisive, analytical mind, and an endless supply of smart ideas, but he still won't make a great leader," Goleman (1998) concluded.

The importance of emotional intelligence goes beyond leadership. David McClelland, PhD, a renowned researcher in human and organizational behavior, found that emotional intelligence also influences performance (McClelland 1998). In 1996, McClelland studied global company Pepsi and found that when senior managers had a critical mass of emotional intelligence, their divisions outperformed annual projections by 20 percent. He also found that division leaders without that critical mass underperformed by the same percentage. His findings were consistent across divisions of the company throughout the world.

EMOTIONAL INTELLIGENCE MATTERS

Travis Bradberry, coauthor of *Emotional Intelligence 2.0*, wrote an article for *Inc.* magazine in 2015 that claimed emotional intelligence scores drop like a rock for those holding director and higher titles, and CEOs have the lowest average emotional intelligence scores in the business world.

But what about the Peter Principle mentioned earlier? Isn't a high level of emotional intelligence more likely to get you promoted than your technical skills? Bradberry agrees that emotional intelligence scores rise steadily from entry-level positions through middle management. Middle managers tend to have high, if not the highest, emotional intelligence scores in the workplace. Most companies would agree that people who are levelheaded and generally good with people should be promoted into management.

Things get interesting, though, when you move past middle management. Emotional intelligence scores decrease dramatically through the director, vice president, and senior executive roles, with CEO at the very bottom.

So how can any CEO be successful? The key to remember is that for each title mentioned in Bradberry's article, the top performers will still be those with the highest emotional intelligence scores. Even though CEOs have the lowest average emotional intelligence scores in the workplace, the best-performing CEOs are those with the highest emotional intelligence scores compared to their counterparts.

Companies that rely solely on business metrics to measure and manage employee performance and make hiring and promotion decisions for positions at any level—entry level to middle management to CEO—will eventually fall victim to the unsustainability of these short-term, bottom-line indicators.

Others in the research and business world agree. Check out this summary from a 2015 *Fast Company* article (Deutschendorf 2015): "Research by the respected Center for Creative Leadership (CCL) in the U.S. found that the primary causes of executive derailment involve deficiencies in emotional competence. Each year, CCL serves more than 20,000 individuals and 2,000 organizations, including more than 80 of the Fortune 100 companies. It says the three main reasons for failure are difficulty in handling change, inability to work well in a team, and poor interpersonal relations."

And, as stated in the *Forbes* article (Jensen 2012): "Research carried out by the Carnegie Institute of Technology shows that 85 percent of your financial success is due to skills in 'human engineering,' your personality and ability to communicate, negotiate, and lead. Shockingly, only 15 percent is due to technical knowledge."

GENDER DIFFERENCES

Goleman (1998) even touches on gender differences in his research. What do you think? Are women more emotionally intelligent than men?

Goleman found that women tend to be more aware of their emotions, show more empathy, and be more adept interpersonally. Men tend to be more self-confident and optimistic, adapt more easily, and handle stress better. His findings were based on averages, though, so any one man might be as good as or better than his female counterpart at being aware of his emotions, and a woman might be as good as or better than her male counterpart at handling stress. Neither set of emotional intelligence qualities is better. Each has its advantages and disadvantages, according to Goleman.

In top business performers, both male and female, the gender differences in emotional intelligence abilities are a wash: Men are as good as women, and women are as good as men.

CAN EMOTIONAL INTELLIGENCE BE LEARNED?

Are truly great leaders born, or are they made? Let's relate this question to you, the emerging healthcare leader. Can you work on developing your emotional intelligence, just as you would your technical skills in our industry? If yes, how would you do that?

According to the *Forbes* article, "Emotional Intelligence . . . is about being aware of your own feelings and those of others, regulating these feelings in yourself and others, using emotions that are appropriate to the situation, self-motivation, and building relationships. Top Tip for Improvement: First, become aware of your inner dialogue. Stress can be a huge killer of emotional intelligence, so you also need to develop healthy coping techniques that can effectively and quickly reduce stress in a volatile situation" (Jensen 2012).

Behavioral therapy demonstrates that change with lasting results requires positive reinforcement over time. People learn best through motivation, extended practice, and feedback. Now that you know the science and research behind emotional intelligence, let's put it into practice.

HOW TO DEVELOP YOUR EMOTIONAL INTELLIGENCE

Now that we've reviewed the supporting research and the business case for emotional intelligence, here are some suggested practices to help you improve your emotional intelligence.

- *Acquire self-awareness.* Remember reading about the importance of self-awareness in chapter 1? Knowledge and awareness of your personality and character—a clear grasp on your strengths and weaknesses, those related to both emotional capabilities and technical skills—may better position you for career advancement. Assessments like StrengthsFinder, Emergenetics, Kolbe, and Myers-Briggs may help in this often-awkward process of self-reflection.

    Laurie tends to be highly instinctive and often is a catalyst for action. She is always ready to engage, which makes her a stellar advisor and project leader, especially when it comes to getting large initiatives off the ground and working under high-pressure deadlines. But the downside of this strength is an impulsive tendency. She responds instinctively from emotion, sometimes without weighing all the consequences of a course of action. For her, with the guidance and feedback of mentors, bosses, and coaches, working on the art of pausing and reflecting before acting has had an incredible impact on her career success. Awareness of the effect of her quick decisions was an area of emotional intelligence that she identified as needing some improvement, and she has worked hard to continue to develop it. To the best of her ability, she has conditioned herself to pause and reflect on situations, to sleep on major decisions, and to seek the counsel of her more deliberative colleagues and advisors before moving forward.

Make reflection a habit. Consistently seek objective information and insight to allow growth and increase self-awareness.

- *Practice self-regulation.* Intentionally prepare for stressful circumstances or those in which you previously reacted in a suboptimal way. Again, set aside time to intentionally reflect on your experiences, and do so frequently. Which recent interactions went well? In which situations were you able to communicate successfully? To negotiate positively or critique someone respectfully? Have you had any meetings or conversations lately that didn't go well? What do you think went wrong? Who seems to push your buttons? Why do you think that is?

  Catalog as many details as you can about the what, why, who, and how related to recent situations that involved working with others. Look for patterns. Assess your progress. Identify blind spots or areas of strength and weakness, set your goals accordingly, and hold yourself accountable for growth.

- *Consistently seek feedback on your performance and the manner in which you engage.* Be open to constructive criticism. If you have a professional mentor or trusted colleagues, ask for their feedback and be open to their candid assessment. Practice seeking and then rationally assessing and acting on the information you receive. Be a good listener. Seek to grow and improve in your leadership of and engagement with those around you. Strive to put yourself in the relationships and social circumstances that position you for maximum success. Be on the lookout for others in your organization whose demeanor or presence you admire. Observe how they carry themselves and navigate challenging circumstances. Learn from them and use their experiences to improve your own performance.

Make an investment in your emotional intelligence. While the concept may be elusive and tricky to measure, its significance to your career success can be far greater than IQ alone. The good news is that, unlike talent and personality, emotional intelligence can be learned and improved.

Often thought of as a soft skill, or a "nice to have," emotional intelligence has a powerful value in the workplace. Talents, skills, and competencies are valuable, but betting on them alone is insufficient. Leaders who achieve the greatest personal and professional success couple technical prowess with emotional and social savvy to influence extraordinary outcomes.

IQ will get you in the door. Emotional intelligence is what will set you apart and allow you to climb the ladder to the highest levels of success and personal well-being.

Remember These

- The greatest challenge of work often involves the human quotient. The emotionally intelligent leader pursues mastery of both the tactical and the human elements of her or his job.

- Research shows that technical skills and cognitive abilities are important drivers of outstanding performance, but considering all three categories as ingredients of success, emotional intelligence is two times more important than the others for job roles at all levels.

→

- Emotional intelligence influences performance. When senior managers in one company had a critical mass of emotional intelligence, their divisions outperformed annual projections by 20 percent. Division leaders without that critical mass underperformed by the same percentage.

- In top business performers, both male and female, the gender differences in emotional intelligence abilities are a wash. Men are as good as women, and women are as good as men.

- Middle managers tend to have high, if not the highest, emotional intelligence scores in the workplace. But when you move past middle management, emotional intelligence scores decrease dramatically through the director, vice president, and senior executive roles, with CEO at the very bottom.

REFERENCES

Bradberry, T. 2015. "Why Leaders Lack Emotional Intelligence." *Inc.* Published March 17. www.inc.com/travis-bradberry/why-leaders-lack-emotional-intelligence.html.

Deutschendorf, H. 2015. "Why Emotionally Intelligent People Are More Successful." *Fast Company*. Published June 22. www.fastcompany.com/3047455/hit-the-ground-running/why-emotionally-intelligent-people-are-more-successful.

Goleman, D. 1998. "What Makes a Leader?" *Harvard Business Review* 76 (6): 93–102.

Jensen, K. 2012. "Intelligence Is Overrated: What You Really Need to Succeed." *Forbes*. Published April 12. www.forbes.com/sites/keldjensen/2012/04/12/intelligence-is-overrated-what-you-really-need-to-succeed/#4d3ae020b6d2.

McClelland, D. 1998. "Identifying Competencies with Behavioural Event Interviews." *Psychological Science* 9 (5): 331–40.

Merriam-Webster. 2017. "IQ." Accessed November 29. www.merriam-webster.com/dictionary/iq.

CHAPTER 4

Pay Attention to Your Character

*Leadership is a potent combination of strategy
and character. But if you must be without one,
be without strategy.*

—*General Norman Schwarzkopf, Jr., former commander
in chief, US Central Command*

Reading Points

- Integrity

- Honesty and Trustworthiness

- Accountability

- Credibility

- How to Strengthen Character

IF A BILLIONAIRE wrote you a $1 million check to spend however you like, how would you treat that check? Would you hold it between your fingers all day long, pass it around to show it off, or leave it unguarded on your desk? Would you risk losing or damaging it? Now consider how you treat something much more valuable than $1 million: your character, something no one can steal from you but that demands more vigilance and protection because ruining it has far greater consequences than destroying a check. Do you pay your character as much attention as you would a huge sum? Do you realize it's equally life changing?

Character is not just a word. It's the entire package of a person's personality, moral and ethical beliefs, motivation, attitude, behavior, thinking and speaking patterns, and so much more. The *Merriam-Webster Dictionary* (2017) defines it as the "way someone thinks, feels, and behaves." Simply put, your character is how those who know you describe your essence to those who don't know you. It's part of your personal brand. (See chapter 6 for more discussion on cultivating your personal brand.)

Of these definitions, the behavior part is, for us, the most important. Why? Because your conduct—including your words—is what people see, feel, interact with, listen and respond to, mimic, and judge. Ultimately, every aspect of your repeated actions over time (and not your intentions, thoughts, feelings, or plans—no matter how noble they are) defines your character in people's minds.

For example, if we say we're committed to our career or organization but consistently miss deadlines, produce sloppy work, don't carry ourselves with decorum, or don't attend events or meetings that contribute to our growth, our behavior shows us to be unreliable at best but untrustworthy at worst. And our reasons for not being able to deliver on our promises? Our bosses don't want to hear those. How about our new pledge to be better? They *really* don't want to hear that.

So watch what you do and what you say at all times. Better yet, be aware of the character (or personality) traits that drive you to behave a certain way. Because as we've said in earlier chapters, knowing your true self is the first step to managing yourself. And the more you manage your character, the more you develop desirable traits, the better you can manage others' perception of you, and the wider you can expand your influence.

In this chapter, we discuss integrity, the building block of good character. It includes the traits of honesty, trustworthiness, accountability, and credibility. These traits are interrelated and build on each other; that is, if you have integrity, you're honest; if you're honest, you're trustworthy; if you're trustworthy, you're accountable; and if you're accountable, you're credible. We also offer tips for properly delivering an apology, caution about practices that could diminish credibility, and strategies for developing character.

But before we get started, let's clarify several points.

1. Character development—like any kind of growth—can be arduous. It requires commitment and self-discipline. (See chapter 5 for more on these concepts.) It requires you to abandon the comfort zone, the status quo, or business as usual. No one else—not us, not your professors, not your mentors, not your bosses, not your peers and coworkers, and not your fairy godmother—but *you* can make that choice or do that work for you. Given that you're reading this book, we think you've made the right choice for your career!

2. Don't wait until you're a titled leader (e.g., a CEO, chief operating office, or vice president) to develop the character-driven qualities that will set you apart from the rest. Start today, if you didn't do it yesterday. Even if your career path or interest changes later, the time and effort you invest in character building will *always* be personally and professionally rewarded. If you're not an early careerist and are already leading people and departments, don't get discouraged and think you're too set in your ways to make adjustments. It's never too late to correct your course or to nurture better habits—regardless of age, job title or level, experience, or industry. Been there, done that? We say, keep doing it!

3. Paying attention to your character is not a one-time process but a lifetime pursuit. It may feel like two steps forward, one step back from time to time. That's natural.

Recovery, learning from it, and applying the lesson to future behavior is part of the process. The different seasons or stages of life—from being a single student to a married, full-time careerist to a retiree—tend to alter some of your character traits. Who you are in your 20s and 30s may not be exactly who you are in your 50s and 60s. Be self-aware enough to notice the differences as you get older and encounter new experiences.

INTEGRITY

Selling out or betraying deeply held convictions for power, monetary gain, or some other benefit. Saying one thing but doing another. Running away from adversity and leaving everyone else to deal with the mess. Lying, misleading, withholding information, blaming someone else, or participating in a cover-up to avoid the consequences of a wrong decision. Associating with or supporting people who are unethical or getting involved in illegal activities. Cheating and committing fraud. These are just some of the behaviors displayed by those who lack integrity. Consider the integrity breaches by "successful" people—from athletes (e.g., professional cyclist Lance Armstrong) to sports coaches (e.g., former Ohio State University football head coach Jim Tressel, former college basketball coach Rick Pitino) to finance titans (e.g., Bernie Madoff) to healthcare administrators (e.g., presidents and CEOs convicted of Medicare fraud and abuse or other legal violations). No amount of wealth, monumental accomplishments, and brilliant skills were enough to save these people from their unscrupulous character. Sure, lacking integrity doesn't stop anyone from attaining their dreams, but it also doesn't help anyone keep living those dreams.

Integrity is the catchall word for being truthful, fair, honorable, ethical, responsible, kind and caring, conscientious, faithful or loyal, and unselfish. In other words, if you have integrity, you do the right thing—all the time, no matter what, regardless of whether anyone is watching. This doesn't mean you always live up to expectations or you don't ever make mistakes. We all make mistakes, of course! But it means you handle each misstep or challenging situation with honesty, humility, consideration of and respect for others' thoughts and feelings, and desire to make things right again. This last point is especially critical because it is about rebuilding trust, the topic of the next section.

There's no better way to illustrate these concepts than to tell a story, so we share a true event that happened to Laurie nearly a decade ago.

Laurie's Apology[1]

I was working on a project with a group of surgeons, a client with whom I had been privileged to work for nearly a decade. Our relationship dynamic was one filled with significant trust and mutual respect. We had lived through an inordinate amount of dysfunction and some unique and harrowing events.

At one point, when I felt that a decision we were leaning toward as a group was not the right one, I took the latitude to go in a different direction. Let me clarify: This was not an operational decision. It did not have significant financial or organizational impact. It was a vendor selection, to be exact.

The group had reached a stalemate in making a decision, mostly due to a personal connection one of the physician-owners had to one of the vendors being considered. In the end, I chose to contract with an alternate vendor, veering away from those we had previously discussed.

When I made this decision, I believed (and still believe) it to be in the best interests of the group. I also knew, without a doubt, that it was going to cause a rift between the physician and me. Taking those factors into consideration, I still moved forward. I alerted the external parties involved, finalized arrangements, and then notified the client of my actions.

As predicted, the physician became very upset. I lost a lot of her trust.

I had built an account of trust with this group, penny by penny and over a number of years. But my decision took a sizable withdrawal from that account. It took a few weeks for the palpable tension between us to wear away and another several months for our relationship to regain the easy stride it once had. Now, eight years later, that event is thankfully a distant memory. But it will always be a distinct learning experience for me.

So how did I come back from that? Slowly but surely, with these simple but powerful acts:

1. *Apologize.* What do you do when you mess up? Do what your mother taught you and say you're sorry. We are not perfect beings, so we make mistakes; those mistakes don't end at some magical point in our career! But no matter how much we err, we shouldn't be too proud to acknowledge our shortcomings and take responsibility for the hurt or damage we caused. It's never fun to apologize, but it's always worth the effort because it reopens the path to communication. (See exhibit 4.1 for further discussion on apology.)

    A brief e-mail exchange followed my original notification to the client, and it was very clear then that the physician was not happy with what I had done. I knew the group's personality and communication style, so I thought it best to apologize in person. Approaching the physicians the next morning to apologize face-to-face was definitely not the easiest thing to do. It was scary! But I knew I needed to show my respect for each of them by looking them in the eye, taking responsibility for my actions, and explaining the thought process behind my decision.

    I didn't apologize because I did something without my client's approval. Again, I still believe my decision was the most appropriate given the circumstances we were in. I apologized because my actions compromised their trust in me. I promised that I would work diligently to regain their trust and restore our relationship, and apologizing was only the first step.

2. *Be humble.* Humility is the natural companion to apology and thus is an essential and nonnegotiable trait of a leader with strong character. If you maintain a humbled approach, you're sending a message that you want to learn and improve from the incident, and the other party's respect for you grows.

    My apology to my client was sincere and humble. Even my written and face-to-face explanations conveyed the tone of my regret. I wasn't defensive or trying to cover up my error; instead, I based my actions on fact and the desire to be helpful. My goal was to walk my client through the steps from beginning to end, without creating a chasm between us. I listened to what they had to say with deference, humbled by their generosity of spirit and the fact that they were willing to give me another chance. This was a valuable learning experience for me. It was a lesson in humility, decision making, and interpersonal relationships all wrapped up into one.

3. *Be honest.* Even in simple situations, it is far better to admit you don't know the answer than to make something up. Politely decline to comment, if you must. But don't engage in a conversation you aren't comfortable having and then dance around the subject because you lack information. Most important, never attempt to cover your tracks. The truth always comes out. The temptation to be dishonest—even if it temporarily lessens the heat on you—is never the right choice.

    During the brief e-mail exchange following the original notification, the physicians asked me several direct questions about what transpired and how I handled certain communications. At least one of those messages was forwarded to other parties, to cross-check or verify my version of the events. Had I not been honest from the start, the situation would have gone from challenging to relationship ending.

Exhibit 4.1 The Art of the Apology

Why is it so hard to apologize? Let's count the reasons:

1. *We're embarrassed.* A mistake of any kind is blush inducing and ego bruising. Apologizing for it only magnifies the error made.
2. *We're afraid to look incompetent.* Will we be seen as weak or not good enough? And if that is the perception, then will it cost us our job, undermine our previous excellent performance, or take away our chances for a promotion?
3. *We're afraid of the risks.* What comes after the apology in which we admit being wrong? Are we legally liable for the fallout? Will it ruin our reputation, our good name? Will it make us a target of jokes, hostility, or retaliation?

Despite these reasons and the high stakes, we have to do the right thing. An apology

- acknowledges the issue and presents an opportunity to right a wrong,

- shows we're human with integrity and humility, and

- starts to restore a damaged relationship.

The qualities of a good apology include the following:

1. *Timely.* Waiting too long is disrespectful. But apologizing too soon doesn't give the receiving party time to react to what happened and thus could prevent them from even processing the apology.
2. *Genuine.* This goes without saying: Don't fake tears, sympathy, empathy, remorse, and other markers of regret and sorrow. Doing so is both obvious and insulting to the receiving party.
3. *Specific.* Address the specific wrongdoing head-on.
4. *Personal.* Approach the other party yourself—no middlemen or messengers allowed. The more personal the delivery is, the better.

(continued)

A face-to-face meeting or a handwritten note always wins over an e-mail or a phone call.

5. *Accountable.* Own up to the wrong, don't pass blame, and don't make excuses.

6. *Educational.* No one is ever too old, too young, too low-level, or too high-level to learn from mistakes, painful experiences, or an uncomfortable apology process and to strive not to repeat them. Learning from the event is the most valuable component of an apology.

Notice that people who are not self-aware and who don't self-reflect tend not to apologize. Is it because of their big egos? Is it because they are so blind to what's going on around them that they don't see the need for an apology? Many of them who do manage to issue an "apology" commit the most counterproductive offenses: (1) pretend the incident never happened, (2) pass the blame, (3) lie, and (4) get defensive.

Master the art of the apology. Because we all make mistakes, it will only be a matter of time until you have to rely on this valuable skill.

HONESTY AND TRUSTWORTHINESS

"Trust is earned a penny at a time and spent in dollar bills." Laurie makes this point each time she speaks to graduate students and emerging leaders about trust. Essentially, it means that trust takes months and years to build but a minute to demolish (although a new school of instant trust has emerged; see Stephen M. R. Covey's book mentioned in chapter 1, for example).

This lesson is evident not only in Laurie's story about her clients but also in Natalie's experiences when she became the new CEO of an established hospital with an existing staff and an involved community (a story shared in chapter 6). We both live by this principle of earning and maintaining trust. How? We conduct ourselves with integrity and approach everything with honesty.

Honesty is not just about telling the truth. It is also about meaning what you say, following through on promises and commitments, presenting the authentic you (not some pretend version), being candid but constructive with your criticism or feedback, not giving false hopes or perceptions by sugarcoating a bad situation, admitting your faults and errors, and practicing transparency. Each time you do something you said you would do (e.g., making a phone call to someone you promised to contact), you are dropping a coin into the other party's trust piggy bank. Each time you share information that would help others improve their job performance or self-understanding, you are dropping a coin into that bank. A lie—even a tiny one—could immediately empty that trust bank. In other words, honesty (not to mention integrity) is the fastest way you can build or break trust.

When you gain people's trust through honesty, they view you as reliable, respectable, accountable, and credible.

ACCOUNTABILITY

We're sure you've heard the phrases "Take responsibility for your actions," "The buck stops here," and "Be part of the solution, not the problem." They all mean the same thing: Be accountable.

Accountability begins with taking ownership of _____ (fill in the blank)—be it a project or assignment, your career trajectory, or your behavior. When you take ownership of a project, for example, you're not merely the person who does your part day in and day out, but you're also the person who pushes yourself to do your part correctly and on time. The phrases "It's not my job" or "I didn't do it" or "I'm on lunch" are not in your vocabulary. You often volunteer to help other team members, and you're honored when someone comes to you for help or advice. You're the first to report your own error in hopes that you could stop it from doing further damage. You admit when you're wrong, don't make excuses but are clear about the reasons, and face consequences graciously. You find finger-pointing ridiculous and punishment unproductive; instead, you value problem solving and not wasting time. And you are a master at being honest with yourself: When something goes wrong, you do a self-assessment to figure out the part you played in the incident so that you don't repeat that gaffe. In a word, when you're accountable, you're committed to, enthusiastic about, and grateful for whatever opportunity or situation you're involved in.

Practicing accountability is not easy because not everything is within our control, and eschewing responsibility is tempting. But your deliberate efforts in this area not only elevate your reputation and add currency to your trust bank but also raise your credibility. The more you showcase that you're accountable, the more you convince others of your credibility—that you can do a job well and deliver great results.

CREDIBILITY

Credibility is a person's level of trustworthiness and believability. Like trust, credibility takes a long time to gain but a short time to lose (see exhibit 4.2). And like trust, it requires maintenance. But unlike trust (which is often measured by the intangible, e.g., integrity and values), credibility is often measured by the tangible (e.g., professional results, accomplishments, and specific skills).

Here's a short list of what makes someone credible:

- Academic or professional credentials
- Work experience
- Trustworthiness
- Transparency
- Accountability
- Strong judgment based on evidence and experience
- Project or organizational outcomes
- Critical thinking and decision-making skills
- Responsiveness and reliability
- Interpersonal abilities and emotional intelligence
- Team orientation

- Expert- or high-level competence
- Workplace and culture savvy
- Advanced social skills
- Focus on goals and results

Now, a word to the wise: Don't get bogged down in definitions. If you Google *difference between trust and credibility*, you'll get millions of results, each seemingly contradicting the others. The important thing to remember is that trust and credibility go hand in hand; no book, article, blog post, or study discusses one without the other. Both are traits that convince people to have faith and confidence in someone's ability. A leader who has a superb character possesses both.

Exhibit 4.2 Eight Ways to Lose Credibility

1. Pass the blame, make excuses, and not take responsibility for your actions
2. Miss deadlines consistently, not follow through, and manage time and priorities poorly
3. Ignore discretion
4. Overpromise and underdeliver
5. Withhold information
6. Participate in or initiate office or organizational gossip
7. Play favorites
8. Pursue or engage in inappropriate personal relationships with a coworker, a boss, a subordinate, or a contractor

---

HOW TO STRENGTHEN CHARACTER

The major and minor actions you take regularly and deliberately define your character. The more you engage in good behavior, the more the behaviors become a habit. The deeper these habits are ingrained in you, the stronger your character and the better your responses to any situation. Identify and then adopt behaviors that exemplify your character, and then embed those behaviors in your daily routine until they become habits.

Exhibit 4.3 presents character-building exercises that you can apply at home, in the office, and anyplace in between.

Exhibit 4.3 Character-Building Exercises

Many of these practices may test your patience and resolve or may feel awkward or like a chore. Those are the feelings you're supposed to have! As Helen Keller said, "Character cannot be developed in ease and quiet. Only through experience of trial and suffering can the soul be strengthened, vision cleared, ambition inspired, and success achieved."

Manage Your Impulses

Do you interrupt or talk over others? Do you make side comments, read your social media feeds, type texts or e-mails, or sigh and yawn audibly when you get bored during meetings or need attention? Do you talk incessantly about yourself to anyone—even complete strangers? Do you throw things, yell, curse, and storm out when you get upset? Do you dismiss people, call them names, or assign them derogatory nicknames? Do you often come to work late, disheveled, and out of it; call in sick; and leave early? If so, are you aware of other people's reactions to you? Are you aware you need to change such behaviors? Why? Because they are untenable, disruptive, disconcerting, unprofessional, and even threatening. If you can't manage your own impulses, you won't be viewed as someone who can manage a staff. When you manage yourself, you are seen as someone who is ready for the next level, someone who can gain people's respect, trust, loyalty, and support.

Invest in Yourself

Read books, volunteer your time and skills, listen to podcasts, follow thought leaders on social media, go to lectures and seminars, travel, meet new people, try new experiences, take a night class. However you decide to invest in yourself, do it often—no matter how busy you get or how uncomfortable you are with the idea—because learning is about challenging yourself and getting to know yourself and so much more in the process. Don't wait for your organization to offer, require, or sponsor a formal continuing education session or program (which you shouldn't miss), but seek and make your own training—however unconventional or informal.

(continued)

Acknowledge Others

Many people in a healthcare facility go unthanked because much of the recognition is focused on the main players—the C-suite, the administrators, the board, the doctors, the nurses, and the other clinicians. But just like in the movies, the bit players often aren't acknowledged because their names are in very tiny print when the credits roll, so to speak. By bit players, we mean the support and maintenance staff whose hard work keeps the facility running smoothly. They deserve to be treated with kindness and respect and to be recognized as a matter of course. Thank them when you can, not just when they've done something for you. Don't ignore them and make them feel invisible, disposable, or less important. Like you, they contribute to the greater goals of the organization. A simple thank-you, nod, hello, smile, quick chat, or just knowing their names would suffice. Leave the generous speeches and pizza parties to your bosses. Beyond this, always give credit where it's due. You've heard that all your life because it's excellent advice.

Practice Hope and Serenity

When you're hopeful, you imbue everything you do with optimism. And when you're optimistic, you tend to be less frazzled and think more clearly—especially in a high-pressure environment like a hospital. And when you're calm amid turmoil, you tend to be perceived as an inspiration and worthy of respect (although people may think you're crazy at first). We know being calm and positive does not seem possible during staff shortages, sweeping layoffs, budget cuts, mergers, and major change initiatives. But diligently trying to remain positive will do much to build your character and boost your own (and others') morale. Plus, "research shows that when people work with a positive mind-set, performance on nearly every level—productivity, creativity, engagement—improves" (Achor 2012).

> ### *Remember These*
>
> - Character is the entire package of a person's personality, moral and ethical beliefs, motivation, attitude, behavior, thinking and speaking patterns, and
>
>   →

so much more. It's how those who know you describe your essence to those who don't know you. It's part of your personal brand.

- Character development—like any kind of growth—can be arduous. It requires commitment and self-discipline. It requires you to abandon the comfort zone, the status quo, or business as usual.
- Don't wait until you're a titled leader to develop the character-driven qualities that will set you apart from the rest.
- Even if your career path or interest changes later, the time and effort you invest in character building will *always* be personally and professionally rewarded.
- Paying attention to your character is not a one-time process but a lifetime pursuit.
- If you have integrity, you do the right thing—all the time, no matter what, regardless of whether anyone is watching.
- Master the art of the apology. Because we all make mistakes, it will only be a matter of time until you have to rely on this valuable skill.
- Trust takes months and years to build but a minute to demolish.
- Practicing accountability is not easy because not everything is within our control, and eschewing responsibility is tempting. But your deliberate efforts in this area not only elevate your reputation and add currency to your trust bank but also raise your credibility.
- Unlike trust (which is often measured by the intangible, e.g., integrity and values), credibility is often measured by the tangible (e.g., professional results, accomplishments, and specific skills).
- Identify and then adopt behaviors that exemplify your character, and then embed those behaviors in your daily routine until they become habits.

NOTE

1.   The original version of Laurie's story appeared at www.
     lauriebaedke.com/2011/02/07/trust-is-earned-a-penny-at-a-
     time-and-spent-in-dollar-bills/. Her story has been edited
     to fit the context of this chapter.

REFERENCES

Achor, S. 2012. "Positive Intelligence." *Harvard Business Review*. Accessed September 1. http://hbr.org/2012/01/positive-intelligence/ar/1.

Merriam-Webster. 2017. "Character." Accessed November 30. www.merriam-webster.com/dictionary/character.

ADDITIONAL RESOURCES

Adams, S. 2014. "Humble CEOs Are Best for Business, New Study Says." *Forbes*. Published July 29. www.forbes.com/sites/susanadams/2014/07/29/humble-ceos-are-best-for-business-new-study-says/.

Biro, M. 2012. "Are You a Character-Based Leader?" *Forbes*. Published September 30. www.forbes.com/sites/meghanbiro/2012/09/30/are-you-a-character-based-leader.

Mixon, E. 2013. "Humility in the Workplace." Published December 11. www.hrtmexec.com/humility-in-the-workplace.

National Public Radio. 2013. "Tact, Tone, and Timing: The Power of Apology." *Talk of the Nation*. Published May 28. www.npr.org/2013/05/28/186922987/tact-tone-and-timing-the-power-of-apology.

Prime, J., and E. Salib. 2014. "The Best Leaders Are Humble Leaders." *Harvard Business Review* Blog Network. Published May 12. http://blogs.hbr.org/2014/05/the-best-leaders-are-humble-leaders.

CHAPTER 5

Consciously Commit to and Exercise Self-Discipline

It takes a deep commitment to change and an even deeper commitment to grow.

—*Ralph Ellison, novelist*

First we make our habits, then our habits make us.

—*Charles Noble, US Army major general and engineer*

Reading Points

- Are You Up for Going All In?
- Why Mind the Little Things?
- What Should You Commit To?
- Strengthening Your Work Ethic
- Strategic Commitment, Not Sacrifice

IF GIVEN A vague promise (I'll call you after the holidays) and a firm commitment (I'll call you on January 3), which would you believe? The former is typically an autopilot response—something you say or do without much thought. The latter, on the other hand, is mindful, intentional, or deliberate—something you've carefully considered and planned. Which group do you belong in?

If you're self-aware, if you practice self-management, and if you pay attention to your character and live with integrity, then you are equipped not only to make a conscious commitment but also to exercise self-discipline. That is to say, you can push yourself, committing to ever-higher goals and then persevering through the inevitable challenges. This combination of commitment and self-discipline (which is every bit a part of your personal brand) applies to everything you do—whether you're training for a grueling 26.2-mile marathon, implementing unpopular or difficult policies and processes, pursuing a certification or an advanced degree, or learning to blend well with the culture of a new organization. Plus, it is an indicator of how strong your work ethic is.

When you commit, you are sending the signal to *everybody* that you are ready for the good, the bad, the ugly, and the unexpected. More important, when you commit, you are sending the signal to *yourself* to use all the resources, techniques, and abilities at your disposal that enable you to deliver on your promise.

In this chapter, we offer practical strategies for helping you commit and apply self-discipline. We also cover the professional areas to which you should commit as well as present a different take on sacrifice, the term often associated with commitment.

ARE YOU UP FOR GOING ALL IN?

If you commit, you have to go all in. And if you go all in, you have to let your conscious mind take over. There are multiple ways to deliberately commit. Here are just a few:

- *Evaluate your psyche.* Why do you want to commit? What motivates or drives you? How determined are you? Are you willing to push through doubt, resistance, setbacks, complications, lack of support, time constraints, exhaustion, pain, illness, hunger, laziness, bad weather, great weather, and anything else that could impede your progress? Do you have enough self-discipline to follow through on plans? Are you a quitter, a finisher, a watcher, or a doer? Which of your character traits will help or hinder you? Self-evaluation should always be the first step in any pursuit, especially a demanding one such as making a commitment. Beyond probing your own psyche, talk to others who know you well. Ask to find out, then listen to learn.

- *Set specific goals—a big one and several little ones.* What do you want to accomplish? When? How? If you get stuck on the details of how, break down the big goal into small but doable parts. For example, if your big goal is to become the director of patient care services two years after earning a master of healthcare administration degree, then your small goals may be finding out the qualifications of the position, honing the relevant skills you already have through on-the-job practice, and acquiring the required skills and experiences through formal and informal education or training. Every goal is a plural; it's composed of many singular objectives, each of which has multiple steps with differing aims. So, when you set a goal, make it as unambiguous as possible. The clearer you are, the better you can articulate a multilayered vision and plan. That detailed goal can be intimidating to pursue, but consider it one of the early tests of your commitment and self-discipline.

- *Make a plan.* Without a plan for how to realize the commitment, you could get sidetracked and quit. Like setting goals, making a plan has to be specific. Specifics may include the steps, time frame, tools and resources, and desired outcomes for each objective and goal. The more details you include, the better your chances of following through on those details (because you don't have to do any guesswork; everything is already laid out). And before you know it, you are living the plan!

- *Track your progress.* If you committed to losing weight, don't you jump on the scale regularly to see whether you're shedding pounds? If you committed to saving money, don't you check your bank balance to see if it's growing? The same idea applies when you commit to professional development, for example. But this time, the measures you use are the feedback from others and the outcomes you've delivered since you first committed to improve. Good or bad or stagnant, the results are informative and could encourage you to try harder or more consciously if you want better outcomes.

- *Make time for what matters.* You designate a time for everything that matters to you, so why not allocate time to allow your commitment to take hold? The time your commitment requires doesn't necessarily have to further complicate or crowd your schedule. Practicing new methods or applying new concepts happens on your feet, or they replace old ones that have become inefficient or ineffective, so they don't take up extra time. And when you scrutinize how you spend your hours during the day, evening, week, and weekend, you likely will find free time for more productive activities. Don't be a cliché and use "too busy" as an excuse; be an original and do the unexpected—make time and make that time count.

WHY MIND THE LITTLE THINGS?

All of the strategies we recommend here and in other chapters can be practiced in increments—a little at a time. There's no set time limit to personal and professional development, and certainly no one is expecting you to completely transform yourself overnight. Many of these strategies take a lifetime to master anyway. Plus, setbacks happen that could undo your progress. So, it only makes sense to take a little-by-little approach.

Self-discipline, much like other character traits, develops one small act at a time. Here's how:

- *Start and finish one task.* Select a task that is simple but not inconsequential or lowest priority, and then set a deadline (e.g., do it for a certain amount of time—like one hour or half a day). Don't let anyone or anything interrupt you (unless, of course, an emergency pops up). Don't think about your other projects. Don't dwell on how many other "better" things you could be doing. Just concentrate on finishing within the deadline. The point of this exercise is threefold: (1) to get you to practice restraint or control your impulse to multitask (multitasking, by the way, is a myth and breeds poor performance because realistically the brain can process only one stimulant at a time), (2) to give you a chance to fully and satisfyingly handle one activity or problem, and (3) to get you to push away thoughts and feelings that weaken your concentration or resolve.

- *Treat yourself.* If you're like us, your work lunch is quick and uneventful; that means no chocolate mousse topped with a swirl of candied fruit or whipped cream for dessert! The things that you enjoy but deprive yourself of—be it dessert, TV time, or some other indulgence—are the very things that you can use as rewards for all your efforts. Self-discipline should not be 24-7 of work and control; it should also be interspersed with celebrations and downtime. The breaks and treats you give yourself represent a pat on the back, gratitude for doing something, an encouragement to continue, and an acknowledgment of the effort—win or lose, goals achieved or not. That's what you'd give to someone else when he has worked so hard and so consistently, right? When you allow yourself the same courtesy, you'll find your mind refreshed and your commitment renewed.

- *Choose carefully.* Admit it: If given five free hours and a choice between watching your favorite show and reading a development book, you'd likely pick the former. That's cool; it's your five hours, after all. But when you consider the time you're devoting to that activity versus the benefits you're gaining from it, you might have second thoughts about that choice. That's the point of our argument: Self-discipline involves the ability to be more discerning about your choices and to remove yourself from tempting situations that might be enjoyable today but could hurt you in the future (Szalavitz 2013). Beware of choices that lead you to slack off. If that's not convincing enough, consider this: Warren Buffett doesn't choose to watch five hours of television every night.

- *Work through the difficulty.* Basketball legend Michael Jordan had the flu but still scored 38 points that led to a Chicago Bulls win during the 1997 NBA finals. *Harry Potter* author J. K. Rowling began writing the wildly popular series while she was on welfare, suffering from depression, and grieving her mother's death. While writing the first edition of this book, Natalie was undergoing onboarding for a new CEO role, while Laurie was immersed in guiding her organization through a merger. There are many more examples of people pushing through seemingly impossible situations and coming out victorious. What these examples tell us is that self-disciplined people don't use adversity, setbacks, and discomfort as an excuse. They persevere, despite their strong impulse to quit, postpone, or forget about the activity they committed to complete or be involved in.

These small acts may seem too minor or too simple to help you become more self-disciplined. But doing them consistently turns them into habits or automatic responses. In turn, the small things add up to huge changes in how you enter into and fulfill a commitment. Jeff Olson (2011, 30), author of the book *The Slight Edge*, said the following about the value of improvement through small acts: "The things you do every single day, the things that don't look dramatic, that don't even look like they matter, do matter. That they not only make the difference—they make all the difference."

WHAT SHOULD YOU COMMIT TO?

We're not telling you what to commit to. That's your job and your choice. What we present in this section are some of the areas that you should commit to improving. Based on our experience, applying a disciplined approach in these areas can help you become the professional who, at least, gets considered for the next opportunity and, at best, gets picked for the next job.

Constant Learning

We hear of an educational seminar or skill improvement training, and we're all ears. We experience a bad day or face a tough situation at work (and at home, too) and automatically ask ourselves what lessons we learned so that we don't repeat it. We didn't get this way because our jobs required it. We didn't get this way because our colleagues or professors or superiors or mentors shamed us into being so. We're both naturally curious, and we're both compelled to become better people and better professionals. We committed to learning long before we decided on what career to pursue, and we never stopped. For us, learning just became a habit, something we don't even think about.

Now let's talk about you.

Did you know job recruiters spend only six seconds to screen each resume? And 80 percent of those six seconds is spent on just a few details, including education (Strom 2013)—the section of your resume that contains not just your degrees but also continuing education or training credits, certifications, and other skill-improvement courses. So, if you want your resume to land in a recruiter's or hiring manager's "yes" pile, beef up the education section.

Beyond what your career requires, you should commit to continual learning to improve you. Here's why:

1. Learning introduces you to innovative ideas, classic and new methods, trends, and different worlds and people. Sure, you might have heard of or even studied some of these things in graduate school, but this type of exposure is hands-on and intended to be more applicable to your current responsibilities and goals. Even if you don't learn anything new (which is unlikely), you'll get a good refresher and come away with a different perspective.

2. Learning gives you an opportunity to network with a diverse group of professionals. Some of these contacts may remain in your life for a long time, serving as resources, business partners, sounding boards, mentors, teachers, or just plain-old friends.

3. Learning widens your view. When you're entrenched in one industry or field, you tend to stick to your kind, speaking the lingo and abiding by the same tried-and-true rules or principles as everyone else. But venturing out of your industry every so often helps you understand how others do their business, manage their staff and operations, and so on. By doing this, you can learn practices that are applicable or even essential to what you do day in and day out. Just look at the process and quality improvement tools that have been adopted in healthcare, such as the Toyota Production System, Six Sigma, and Crew Resource Management (from the automobile, electronics, and aviation industries, respectively) or the term *customers* or *consumers* now applied to patients (from the for-profit sector and the marketing industry).

Thanks to the Internet and advancements in technology, constant learning is now easier than ever to commit to. Learning options include YouTube and Vimeo channels, podcasts, blogs and vlogs, on-demand streaming, webinars, and audiobooks and e-books (which Laurie prefers) on top of in-person lectures, seminars, conferences, and meetings (which Natalie prefers). Find out which format works best for you, pick a subject (if it's a one-topic, one-class arrangement) you are interested in or need to boost or acquire skills in, devote the time to it, and sign up or attend. Beyond these ideas, we also suggest reading management and leadership books written for a general audience. Check out books by Jim Collins, Patrick Lencioni, Brené Brown, and Adam Grant, to name just a few.

If you continue to learn, you could become that rare person who is knowledgeable about a lot of things *and* an expert in one thing. That is an asset no one can take away from you.

Building Relationships

Many kinds and levels of relationships exist in healthcare, and all of them are important. Your commitment in this area is not just about creating connections (through networking, mentorship, fellowship/internship, and normal business operations) but also nurturing and maintaining those connections by serving them.

We've mentioned before that your connections are a good resource. You may ask them to give you feedback, advice, support, opinions, and other business-related favors. But let us clarify this notion.

Do so only *after* establishing a rapport with your connections, and always focus on what you can do for them or how you can serve them—not the other way around. Although almost every relationship ultimately yields a mutual benefit for the parties involved, the benefits shouldn't be the only reason you are forging a connection with someone. When you do gain some kind of benefit, pay it back by not letting down those who reached out to you or pay it forward by becoming a mentor or opening doors for someone else.

Committing to building relationships means performing the small acts of meeting new people, finding a commonality, getting to know each other over time, treating others with kindness and respect, calling or e-mailing once in a while to say hello or ask about their life, offering help without an expectation of a favor in return, sending handwritten notes and cards when appropriate, and even visiting when the other is in town. This kind of nurturing takes years—perhaps even decades. It's a true manifestation of self-discipline.

Even a mentor–mentee/protégé relationship requires some TLC. Mentors are not fairies who grant favors and make wishes come true. They are teachers and advisors who dispense knowledge and insights—voluntarily. The wisdom and understanding you gain by listening to them are the cake and icing, so to speak; anything beyond that is decoration. They really don't owe you anything.

If you don't have a mentor, approach someone whose character, style, and achievements are admirable to you. If you do have a mentor, acknowledge that person's contributions to your growth and express your gratitude—not just once but regularly.

Asking for Help

Asking for help means admitting to your boss that you didn't understand the directives for your new assignment. It means getting verification straight from the source of information—even if that person is a member of the C-suite or the board—to ensure you don't end up wasting valuable resources. It means networking with like-minded professionals who are facing the same challenges as you are. It means accepting assistance from those who have more experience and knowledge.

What it *doesn't* mean (or shouldn't make you feel) is that you're incompetent or inadequate. In fact, asking for help is a sign that you're self-aware and open to opportunities and new ideas. It also shows you are so committed to your job and career that you're willing to go to great lengths to get things right. The flip side to not asking for help is isolation. Isolation—from learning, networking, and improvement opportunities—is perhaps one of the worst situations you can find yourself in at any time, but especially when you're building a career.

Thinking Outside the Box

We know this is cliché, but don't discount it. Being innovative is not just for Silicon Valley. It pays off in other industries, too. Take, for example, the story of how Natalie found one of her mentors. Every Friday, her graduate program invited CEOs to speak to the students. Afterward, the students had an opportunity to meet the CEO and ask follow-up questions. Natalie went beyond talking and shaking hands with the CEOs. She handed each of them her business card stapled to her resume, introduced herself, and asked, "Can I take you to lunch? Can I pick your brain?"

It was a bold move, but it didn't always yield the results she wanted. Although many CEOs said yes, most never called. In fact, as she was leaving one of those sessions, she found her resume with her business card in the trash can—right outside the room! Disappointed, embarrassed, but not beaten, Natalie picked it up and continued her plan. After all, there were more Fridays to come and more CEOs to meet.

And then she met her future mentor, a well-known healthcare leader who has consistently been named as one of *Modern Healthcare's* 100 Most Influential People in Healthcare. When she gave this leader her quick spiel, he said yes. She was overjoyed because she'd always admired him. And when his assistant called her 30 days later to set up a lunch meeting at one of the nicest restaurants in town, she was floored. Twelve years later, Natalie continues to meet with that mentor for lunch twice a year. Their mentoring relationship has flourished and has been fully rewarding.

Healthcare management is a competitive field, so get creative with your approach to stand out from the crowd. If you get more nos than yeses, more doubters than believers, so what? Take that calculated risk. But whatever strategic move you make, ensure that it is always professional, always appropriate, and never too over the top that you're attracting the wrong kind of attention.

STRENGTHENING YOUR WORK ETHIC

A strong work ethic shares the same DNA with strong character. That is, if your work ethic is superb, you take ownership of your performance and results, you care about the quality of your work, you're a team player but capable of working independently, you're honest about your knowledge and skills, and you do more than what the assignment or project requires. In other words, you have integrity that enables others to trust you as well as deem you responsible and credible.

A commitment to strengthening your work ethic requires both self-discipline and mental discipline. We're not going to discuss the intricacies of mental discipline here, but suffice it to say that if self-discipline is *how hard* you work, then mental discipline is *how well* you work. When you're mentally disciplined, you are in control of how you think about and respond to situations and you can choose to be positive rather than negative.

Some of the small acts you could do to boost your work ethic include the following:

1. *Change your attitude.* You may be the hardest worker around, but if you're grumpy, negative, or disengaged, you may not find willing volunteers or helpers for your projects. No one wants to work with an unhappy person

or someone with a chip on her shoulder. Not only is attitude contagious, but it can also hamper your career.

2. *Manage your time.* If you know you tend to procrastinate or get distracted easily, start your projects early and ask for an extension as soon as necessary. Missing a deadline is understandable if it happens only sometimes. But if it happens all the time, it will affect not only the types of projects you are assigned but also your professional reputation. The worst thing you can do is make excuses or rationalize why you are late. Own up to your mistake and apologize. And do not let it happen again.

3. *Be strategic.* See the next section.

STRATEGIC COMMITMENT, NOT SACRIFICE

When you commit to developing your career, you may not realize what it entails until you're neck-deep into it. For example, you may know that studying for the American College of Healthcare Executives (ACHE) Board of Governors Examination in Healthcare Management will take a lot of time, but you may not know that it could take 10 to 15 hours a week. That's a huge chunk of time away from your loved ones, your hobbies, and anything else that matters to you. Of course, as we've said over and over again, you have a choice: Put in the hard work and enjoy the long-term benefits, or opt out and enjoy the short-term relief but suffer the long-term consequences.

There is no shortcut to personal and professional growth. No quick fix. No magic wand. But there is such a thing as changing your mind-set so that you view the work involved not as a painstaking sacrifice but rather as a conscious strategic commitment. Take Laurie's story, for example.

As a young professional, Laurie left a healthcare executive job to launch her own consulting practice. She wanted the time flexibility that the business afforded her so that she could be present for her husband and young children yet continue to fulfill her professional aspirations as an industry leader and entrepreneur. Although technically she gave things up—such as a guaranteed paycheck, a collegial team environment, daily access to colleagues and superiors, and the support and resources of an established organization—she never saw those losses or her decision as a sacrifice. Instead, she deemed the move as a strategic choice or commitment.

Laurie went on to pursue board certification from both ACHE and the American College of Medical Practice Executives, giving up months' worth of time to study for board exams and write case studies and an academic paper. Her strategic commitment paid off. She earned the certifications, a distinction that fewer than 15 percent of her contemporaries in the industry possess. She built a national speaking practice, becoming a frequent keynote presenter at state Medical Group Management Association chapter conferences, a recurring faculty member at the annual ACHE Congress on Healthcare Leadership, and a facilitator of physician and leadership development programs for healthcare organizations nationwide.

What if you, too, started looking at decisions in your life as strategic commitments (gains) rather than sacrifices (losses)? Start small.

Say you commit to growing your network but you don't have time to attend networking events. You don't have to sacrifice a Saturday or Sunday or even a weeknight to do that; you could network during lunch. Instead of dining with your regular lunch group every day, once or twice a week have lunch with people you want to network with. This way, you not only keep your set of work friends but also gain new associates.

Changing your mind-set, changing your attitude, making conscious or strategic decisions, turning negatives into positives—whatever you want to call it, it works. It's a part of the framework of commitment and self-discipline. Go ahead and give it a try!

Rookie Mistakes

Coasting

It's easy to coast through a job when you're just starting out. No one is expecting you to shoot straight to the C-suite. No one is pressuring you to go back to school to update your skills. No one is giving you complicated or high-traffic departments to run on your own. And that's precisely why you shouldn't be complacent. You have to take control of your career early and always. If you don't, you could remain under the radar. Commit to advancing your career, and do the difficult work necessary to prove that commitment.

Being Tactical Instead of Strategic

Eric was an administrative fellow in a health system. One day, he volunteered to take and then distribute the minutes for senior management meetings—meetings he had no reason to be in. His mentor, the president, agreed. Eric found the task tedious and unglamorous . . .

Let's stop here for a pop quiz: Did Eric make a mistake? Yes, no, maybe? Why? This is not an open-book quiz, so don't look ahead to the rest of the story.

. . . but it afforded him unparalleled access to the inner workings of the system and allowed him to build stronger relationships with key executives. The experience was incredibly valuable to Eric's career development.

What was your answer? Did you guess how the story ended? How?

Healthcare is replete with true stories like this. This one demonstrates the value of being strategic rather than tactical.

→

When you're tactical, you think in terms of the here and now (the short term). When you're strategic, you think of the far and away (the long term). The problem with being tactical is that it doesn't allow you a view of the big picture. And if you fail to see the big picture, you miss out on unique and strategic opportunities that offer great rewards. Change your mind-set and start to make conscious, strategic moves. Then, create and share your own success story.

Staying Isolated

When you land your first healthcare job, learn the ropes of your new position, and get comfortable with the idea of busy professionals of all types consulting and commiserating with you, you may start to think that there's no more need to try, that you have found the tribe you belong with for the rest of your career, and that networking is a thing of the past. But you'd be wrong. It's good to make connections with people at work, but it's also worthwhile to expand your reach to people outside your immediate circle. After all, you might want to change careers, organizations, or industries later. The more relationships you build now, the greater the likelihood that those people will be there to support you later.

Remember These

- Conscious commitment is the voluntary, mindful dedication to something.
- Self-discipline involves the ability to be more discerning about your choices and to remove yourself from tempting situations that might be enjoyable today but could hurt you in the future.

→

- Self-disciplined people don't use adversity, setbacks, or discomfort as an excuse. They persevere, despite their strong impulse to quit, postpone, or forget about the activity they committed to.

- Small, disciplined acts when practiced consistently turn into habits or automatic responses. In turn, the small things result in huge changes in how you enter into and fulfill a commitment.

- Gaining benefits shouldn't be the only reason you are forging a connection with someone.

- To be highly productive and highly successful in your line of work, you have to do what's necessary. And often what's necessary is difficult and frustrating and demanding.

- Self-discipline is *how hard* you work, while mental discipline is *how well* you work. When you're mentally disciplined, you are in control of how you think about and respond to situations and you can choose to be positive rather than negative.

- There is no shortcut to personal and professional growth. No quick fix. No magic wand. But there is such a thing as changing your mind-set so that you view the work involved not as a painstaking sacrifice but rather as a conscious strategic commitment.

REFERENCES

Olson, J. 2011. *The Slight Edge: Turning Simple Disciplines into Massive Success*, revised edition. Lake Dallas, TX: Success Books.

Strom, D. 2013. "What Recruiters Look for in a 6-Second Resume Scan." *Dice.* Published June 9. https://insights.dice.com/2013/01/09/what-recruiter-look-for -in-a-6-second-resume-scan.

Szalavitz, M. 2013. "Self-Disciplined People Are Happier (and Not as Deprived as You Think)." *Time.* Published June 24. http://healthland.time.com/2013/06/24/ self-disciplined-people-are-happier-and-not-as-deprived-as-you-think.

ADDITIONAL RESOURCE

Hoffmann, W., M. Luhmann, R. R. Fisher, K. D. Vohs, and R. F. Baumeister. "Yes, but Are They Happy? Effects of Trait Self-Control on Affecting Well-Being and Life Satisfaction." *Journal of Personality* 82 (4): 265–77.

Building and Maintaining a Forward-Moving Career

In part I, we covered the foundational concepts and approaches for developing you—the way you conduct yourself, interact with and influence others, and do your work—so that you can stand head and shoulders above the rest. In part II, we pull from these basics and expand our discussion to include strategies and tactics that help you build and grow a career in the competitive and challenging field of healthcare management.

Specifically, we address why it's important to curate (read: be intentional about) what you share on social media and why it's advisable to match your online brand to your authentic offline persona. We also talk about understanding what you're doing (performance), how you're doing it (style), and how that style could help or hamper both. Plus, we explain the principle of servant leadership, a model focused on the others instead of the self; the inevitability of failures; the art of forming and nurturing relationships (aka networking); and the importance of finding and becoming a mentor.

Our goal in these chapters is to emphasize that career building and maintenance is not a solitary, stable pursuit, but rather an activity that relies on other people and involves many ups and downs. Don't want to police your behavior, take risks, reach out to others, try new things, fail every once in a while, and serve your stakeholders? Then expect to be stuck, to find yourself in the same spot year after year while your peers move on and up. When you read the Note to My 25-Year-Old Self features distributed throughout this book, you'll see that our recommendations are echoed by the same people who have led and still are leading the field today.

Note to My 25-Year-Old Self

When I was 25, I was married with a 15-month-old baby, and my wife was pregnant with our second child. Needless to say, this was an incredibly significant and defining time in my life. I was completing my bachelor's degree in medical technology and driving a long distance in the wee hours of the morning for my internship. My wife was teaching school, and the process of juggling our daily activities was, to say the least, a challenge! As I look back on those times, I wonder how these life experiences were helping me to prepare for my future and how I was looking at them to help me to develop my leadership skills and traits.

I am blessed to have been surrounded by incredible mentors, leaders, and just good people whom I was able to seek out and have conversations with about where I was and where I wanted to go with my future. Most important in that group was my wife. She was the confidant I needed to share my hopes and aspirations with; the one who gave me an unjudging kick in the pants to get going when I needed it; and, most important, the person I could talk to about my fears and occasional lack of confidence. All of us, at some time, need a special mentor and confidant who acts as a listening post and guide in our lives. As I have gotten older, and hopefully a bit wiser, I have found that my need for this type of help and advice has grown and not diminished. It has been through these precious relationships that I have been able to overcome adversity and find new ways of looking at challenges I have faced in my career and in life. My advice to you is to consistently and intentionally seek relationships and counsel with mentors and others who can offer valuable advice and accountability, to groom you for continued growth.

So why is this important? As a 25-year-old, I often thought I knew all the answers and how to get from point A to point Z in the most efficient and effective manner. What I have learned is that I didn't know anything! In fact, I was missing many of life's opportunities to learn by not stopping at point B or C or D. I was rushing through life so fast that I was missing out on the richness of the journey. I wanted to get on with life so I could become something I wasn't at that time. But it has been my observation that my life and career, and those of others in my line of sight, are not necessarily linear. Expect setbacks and detours. Be patient. Be open to learn from the process. And embrace the journey.

A mentor once told me I should consider establishing a personal mission statement. I did so, and to this day I've worked to use it as a reference for decision making in my personal and professional life. It has helped me to remember who I am and the virtues, abilities, and habits I have committed to, and to continually work to improve myself so I can achieve the potential I have been given. I encourage you to do the same. Spend time reflecting on your purpose and the values and beliefs that you hold dear. Clarify them, and revisit them periodically. They will be a powerful and effective filter in your future decision making.

Now, some 35 years later, it is my privilege to be a mentor, a confidant, and a listening post to the 25-year-olds who are beginning their professional journeys in our noble profession. I see the value of having curated relationships with those who had varied perspectives and paths in their personal and professional life. Coming to realize that you do not know it all is a first step in becoming a great leader. Acknowledging that you need to reach out to others to gain diverse perspectives, and to seek coaching and encouragement, demonstrates that you are gaining maturity and wisdom.

My definition of leadership is providing an environment and culture that allow people to rise to their highest potential, looking at people not as who they are but as who they can become. As a

25-year-old, I would want to place myself in an environment where my potential could be cultivated by trusted leaders, mentors, and advisors. A place where my priorities could be established. And a place where I could experiment and enjoy the journey from A to Z while benefiting from the rich experience it offers.

Signed,
Edward H. Lamb, FACHE
Chairman (2016–2017), American College of Healthcare Executives
President and CEO, Mount Carmel Health System

CHAPTER 6

Cultivate Your Personal Brand

Your brand is what people say about you
when you're not in the room.

—*Jeff Bezos, founder, Amazon.com*

Reading Points

- Finding the True You

- Curating Your Online Posts

- Maintaining Professional Decorum

- Networking on Social Media

NAME A BRAND, any brand. Did you name your favorites? Did you name yourself? Are you aware that you are a brand as well?

A personal brand is all about what an individual represents and how that image is perceived. Specifically, your brand includes your name, gender, occupation, character, education and training, personal and professional style (including leadership style; see chapter 7), skills and talents, accomplishments, associations, and reputation. If you're on social media, your brand is represented by your posts; photos; status updates; comments or responses; things you "like," favorited, or upvoted; tags; links shared or forwarded; and following and follower lists. These are the details people associate with your brand—both offline (or "in real life") and online. Like consumer brands, your personal brand elicits conscious and subconscious reactions from anyone who meets, talks to, or hears about you. If these people were playing a word-association game, what do you think they'd say when your name comes up?

Keep your offline and online personas consistent with each other. That is, be aware of the discrepancy between who you are in real life and who you seem to be on the computer screen. Contradictions between the two often send the message that you're not being your authentic self. For example, if friends, family, coworkers, and bosses know you as a caring, intelligent individual, they will be shocked and dismayed if you tweeted something that bullies or shames anyone—whether in a personal or professional context. Don't confuse and surprise your audience, as they have the power to tarnish your brand—that is, if your own behavior doesn't tarnish it first.

In this age of do-it-yourself everything, the web has become the number-one tool for finding information about a person. Even if you're not an active web user, you still have an online presence. What will a simple Google search of your name reveal about your brand? Will it turn up your social media accounts? Awards and achievements? Embarrassing posts or pictures? Good or bad, the answers are the reason you should continually cultivate your personal brand. The better you are offline, the better you'll look online.

This chapter offers the dos and don'ts of cultivating your brand. As usual, we present examples, recommendations, and tips.

FINDING THE TRUE YOU

Self-awareness, the result of self-reflection, is the first multilayered step to cultivating your brand (see chapter 1). When you have a strong grasp of who you are, you can better manage and improve your interactions and relationships, your self-development needs, others' expectations of and reactions to you, your influence on others, and so on. Equally important is that you become more authentic, aware of your abilities and accomplishments but at the same time humbled by your limitations, weaknesses, and work-in-progress status. This kind of authenticity is important to your brand because it makes you relatable.

Although we addressed self-awareness strategies extensively in chapter 1, we review some small-act tips here:

- *Step outside yourself.* How do you see yourself? How do you think others see you? What types of people do you attract and what types attract you, and why? Would you hire or fire someone like you, and why? Do your activities and behavior in and out of work embarrass or inspire others? Do you edit parts of yourself or your experiences in discussions or conversations, and why or why not? Which things about you are you proud to tell others, and which would you rather keep to yourself? Have others criticized you in the past, and what did you do with that information? What one word would your coworkers or bosses use to describe you? These questions will trigger other probing questions. Answer them honestly; you don't have to report your findings to anyone, but you do have to act on them.

- *Ask a friend, family member, coworker, or mentor to be honest about you.* Give them permission to be as candid as possible, and reassure them that their opinions will not affect your relationship (although they could hurt your feelings). Try not to be defensive about the details they bring up; they are not attacking you but giving you much needed feedback. And that feedback could range from how you communicate verbally, in writing, and with your body (Do you speak clearly? Are your e-mails, papers, tweets, reports, and texts riddled with typos and/or slang? Do you look people in the eye? Is your handshake firm?) to how you conduct yourself professionally (Do you show up late to meetings? Do you pay attention or listen without distractions? Is your attire business appropriate? Are you reliable and do you take responsibility for your mistakes?) to what attitudes you typically display (Are you an optimist or a pessimist? Do you welcome or avoid change? Are you snarky and sarcastic or compassionate and sensitive?).

- *Make a list of what makes you uniquely you.* List your beliefs, likes and dislikes, talents, skills, character traits, behavioral tendencies, achievements and failures, types of people you associate with, personal and professional goals, activities or causes you participate in, and any other components that define who you are.
- *Review your online and offline activities.* Your social network profiles, comments on various sites, blog posts, tweets, posted pictures and videos, and all other activities on the web don't exist in a vacuum. The same goes for offline activities. Knowing what you spend your time on is a good step to understanding the *you* brand.

Revisit these small acts periodically. Invest time quarterly or annually to take stock of your growth. Be honest. Be intentional. And remember that what gets measured, gets managed.

One caveat: Although you should embrace (and celebrate) your authentic self, you must consider how it affects those around you. Be careful about (or even change) the aspects of you that could potentially cause more harm than good to your brand, especially when displayed online, where it's hard to retract what you say and do.

CURATING YOUR ONLINE POSTS

In the years before Facebook and Twitter (gasp!), defining your personal brand meant how you conducted yourself at networking events and what catchphrase was written on your business card. If you wanted your brand to take a slightly different direction or if you made a mistake, no problem! All you had to do was change your strategy or behavior going forward, and all was well. That's not as true today because most of us now work and play on the web, where all our personal and professional actions and decisions can be viewed with a quick search—even if we don't use our real name.

If you're a 24-year-old master of healthcare administration (MHA) graduate, for example, and you've been on Facebook since you were 15, guess what? Your status updates from nine years ago—when you were still in high school—are just as much a part of your personal brand as your Facebook activities today. Same goes for old photos, old videos, and old comments you shared online. Scary, but true.

Our point is not to scare you, though. We're here to remind you that what is posted today will be around for a long time—most likely permanently. Juvenile activities could harm your brand and thus your chances for a huge promotion, an interview for a dream job, or any other once-in-a-lifetime opportunity. It's no secret that employers put on their sleuthing caps and search the web for any (negative and positive) information on a prospective or current employee.

Although you can't do anything about the past, you can control what you do today. Err on the side of caution and agonize too much, rather than too little, over a post instead of letting everything fly without considering the consequences or the blow to your brand. Avoid such consequences with these three basic but self-disciplined steps:

1. *Review your privacy settings.* You can adjust how much of your social media profiles your family members, friends, colleagues, and the general public can see or access. But remember this: Even with the most conservative or restrictive privacy settings, that inappropriate photo or post you or someone else uploaded can still find its way into the hands of employers and those who can make your shame viral. You could pay huge amounts of money for a reputation management company to sweep the web of all the negative images and posts related to you, but this effort may not be enough.

2. *Filter yourself.* As we mention repeatedly, self-awareness—along with self-discipline—is critical. The more aware you are of how others perceive you (and the implications of those perceptions), the more likely you will think before posting. For each status update, comment, tweet, or photo upload, ask yourself: Does this really align with the professional image I want to project? Or more simply: Will I regret this? When in doubt, leave it out.

3. *Bite your tongue.* Never, ever speak ill of your job, colleagues, and employers. Online, everything and everyone should be regarded as great. Your job is a dream. Your colleagues are fantastic. Your boss is the best ever. Your workplace can't be beat. While in some cases these statements may not be true, online is not the place to air your dirty laundry. We're not suggesting that you lie, but rather that you should not burn bridges or disregard people's feelings. If you would not say negative and hurtful words to anyone to their face or within their earshot, then you should not type disparaging comments about anyone online. The two are essentially the same thing. If you must (for some reason) include the people and the place that employ you in your conversation, don't complain. No matter how cryptic, witty, or disguised your criticism is, it

can be identified and can get back to those you're targeting. Depending on your company's social media policy, you may be handed a box of your belongings and escorted from the building the next time you show up to work.

No matter their role or rank, no one is too valuable to be fired. Even owners, board chairs, and CEOs can fall, and have fallen, into this trap. So be careful what you say out there!

MAINTAINING PROFESSIONAL DECORUM

Wear professional business attire, be well groomed, and maintain good personal hygiene. Modulate your voice, enunciate, articulate, don't use words you don't fully understand, and keep slang to a minimum—or better yet, don't use slang at all. Don't slouch, keep your chin up, firmly shake hands (don't crush or jerk), and look people in the eye. Show confidence, humility, respect, and gratitude. Do all these things when you first meet people, during official work functions, and in job interviews. We know we sound like a drill sergeant, but this is an important message that we must deliver directly. Professional decorum elevates the *you* brand; no one will dispute that. And as we say in our sessions, carry yourself *as if* you are already filling the job of your dreams.

Looks Matter

Let's talk about your appearance—specifically, the way you dress and the way you present to others. In the modern, more sensitive world we live in, it's almost taboo to talk about judging people based on looks. But let's be realistic—it happens, even if we don't intend for it to happen. The blind-audition portion of the popular TV show *The Voice* gives aspiring singers a chance to showcase their abilities to a panel of superstar judges whose backs are turned so that they cannot see the performers. The contestants focus on singing and nothing else because they know they are only going to be judged on their voice, not their appearance. Unfortunately, the rest of society does not work like *The Voice*.

People do judge you for how you look, and the sooner you accept that, the better off you'll be. Professionals have long held that it takes only a few minutes to make a first impression on someone, while others argue that we get only about 30 seconds. Author Malcolm Gladwell (2007) claims that impressions are made even faster—one to two seconds maximum. You have only those quick seconds to make as strong a first impression as possible and to judge or make up your mind about those who are standing in front of you.

Again, assessing your appearance comes back to self-awareness. Look in that mirror and be honest about what message you are sending. Better yet, ask friends for their frank assessment. You might love your personal style (e.g., trendy clothes and accessories, colorful hair, visible piercings and tattoos), but consider how that style translates in a professional, formal environment. What message is it sending to a job recruiter or a future boss, and how is it tainting their perception of you? They don't yet know that beneath the style (which might intimidate some people) is an incredibly smart, creative, capable, and hardworking you. It's their loss, right? Wrong. It's your lost opportunity—and a preventable loss at that.

Every work environment or culture operates by a set of rules, including the dress code. When you are trying to fit in or dress appropriately, you have to match your appearance with that of everyone else in the organization. For example, if everyone (including the CEO) at your small, rural community hospital wears khakis, cotton shirts, and loafers, you ought to dress in the same way. How will you relate to them if you show up in a pinstriped suit and designer shoes every day? The opposite is also true. If your board members always wear formal professional attire (i.e., suit and tie for men; dress suit or pantsuit for women), then you should do the same on the day you're meeting with or presenting to them—even if the outfit is not what you wear to work daily. If you're meeting with the property maintenance team for a once-a-year, all-day logistics strategy session for the organization's big annual events, show up in jeans and a T-shirt branded with the hospital logo— just like the team members wear all the time. Dressing according to the accepted style of a work group or the culture helps you gain instant acceptance and earn trust, regardless of whether your coworkers realize that is what's happening.

For example, Anna worked in a hospital's information technology department. She was one of a handful of women who worked among a throng of male computer programmers. The environment was jeans-only, so for the first few days on the job, she showed up in skinny jeans and high heels. She looked like a knockout. The programmers, on the other hand, struggled to keep their unironed shirts tucked into their ill-fitting jeans. Needless to say, the men were intimidated by her. Anna soon realized this, though. When she returned to work wearing relaxed-fit jeans and flats, she found that her ability to communicate effectively with the programmers suddenly improved.

The point is that managing your personal self (personality and style included) and your professional self (leadership style included) takes a fine balance. Work is not always the appropriate place to express your true personality, especially if you are a newcomer. You often have to conform your personality (in this case, your appearance) to the environment, not the other way around. That is not to say that your personality—which is a strong part of your personal brand and the first piece of that brand people notice— should be locked out of the workplace. How much or how little of your personality to take with you is up to you. But be aware that, in the professional setting, you must make sure your personal brand sends the message you want to convey. The same is expected of you on social media.

NETWORKING ON SOCIAL MEDIA

With today's social media, there has never been an easier time to build your personal brand. Instead of only being able to network at in-person gatherings—such as your health administration program's sponsored events or a healthcare association's annual conference (e.g., the American College of Healthcare Executives [ACHE] Congress on Healthcare Leadership)—you can also network online. And you can do it efficiently and effectively. Just like networking in person, networking online isn't about meeting someone and immediately asking for the "sale." It's about getting to know people and building relationships—relationships that can provide mutual benefits for months and years down the road.

How to get started? Establish an account on LinkedIn and Twitter, for example. Scan or search for thought leaders on your topics of interest. Who are the favorite authors, speakers, or bloggers in your industry or other related fields? Who are prominent executives from your organization, your community, and your profession? Follow them, as well as associations, publications, or organizations whose work relates to your work, your interests, or your aspirations. On Twitter, you may search using hashtags to find information and contributors by topic (e.g., #leadership, #innovation, #patientsafety) or using the monikers promoted by specific conferences or events (e.g., #ACHECongress).

The number-one mistake professionals make online is failing to remember that interacting and networking on the web requires the same respect and the same decorum as interacting and networking face-to-face. The second biggest mistake? Forgetting that online, everything is visible and everything is permanent, as we mentioned earlier. If you conduct yourself *as if*, you should be fine.

We're not going to list social media sites and how they can help you network. Because the web and technology are ever advancing, sites and applications change quickly. Keep tabs on online networking trends throughout your career. For now, Twitter, Facebook, and LinkedIn are the most popular among professionals. Our recommendation is to use Facebook for personal, LinkedIn for professional, and Twitter for a blend of the two.

Dedicating each site to a specific use is a good way keep your message consistent in each platform. For example, if you regularly share healthcare-related news, MHA class information, and other helpful industry or career resources on LinkedIn, then your networks or connections know that you are on the site for professional or business purposes. Don't suddenly switch to discussing the best chili recipes—save that for Facebook! If you are using Twitter for both personal and professional purposes, make sure that you maintain professional decorum, even though you may not always be tweeting about work. Keep it clean (including being selective about whom you follow and which posts you retweet), as you are representing the *you* brand to all your followers.

When networking online, you must be self-aware, smart, and authentic. You must also be cautious. Be cognizant of the fact that you are not just the main face of your personal brand but also an indirect representative of your current organization—even if you aren't the organization's official spokesperson, publicist, or account/profile administrator. If the organization is listed on your resume, bio, or CV as your employer, then your words and actions reflect upon that company. Take that responsibility seriously.

We saved the best for last: Offline and online, the more defined your personal brand, the more value it holds. As you progress in your career and if you continue to improve yourself and cultivate your brand, you won't need to search endlessly for greater roles and new opportunities. Those things will come to you. Your brand will speak for itself, your robust network will support you, and you will get offers. For now, you have work to do.

Rookie Mistakes

Tweeting Like No One's Watching

Several years ago, during an industry conference, Laurie stumbled on a tweet by another attendee. The tweet was a pleasant, professionally composed compliment to the organization that put together the conference. Laurie was quite impressed with the message, so she decided to click on the name of the attendee to find out more. He turned out to be a new MHA graduate looking for his first job in healthcare. Laurie then scrolled down to read his other tweets, and soon wished she hadn't. His past tweets (some as recent as two days before the conference) were full of foul language, rude and arrogant remarks, and other not-safe-for-work musings. And they were all public, for the world to see. Laurie doesn't know what became of him; all she knows is that she could never endorse, hire, or network with someone as self-*un*aware as he was.

Dressing for the Nightclub

Natalie once interviewed for a very competitive job. All the candidates were highly accomplished. One (let's call him Joe) had qualifications that mirrored those of Natalie. He was a sprint runner in college, just like her. And he even taught middle school, just as she did. On interview day, Joe wore a nice suit—and a colorful printed shirt with no tie. In fact, his shirt was open to reveal an undershirt. His hair could use a comb, and his shoes could be a lot less pointy. Frankly, he looked like he just got home from the club. After a long day of interviews, Natalie got the job.

→

To be fair, Joe didn't land the job *merely* because of what he looked like. But his appearance certainly didn't win him points. Perhaps had he shown up in professional attire, the interviewers might have viewed him as a more serious contender and might not have been too quick to eliminate him from the tight competition. The small details of his appearance—especially the opened, printed shirt—were not just distracting but also sent a clear message that his head was not in the game and he was not ready for the next level. When your life and career are on the line, why let anything get in the way of your success? Dress your best, show up on time, and be as prepared as you possibly can be. You cannot do a thing about how the competition shows up, but you can certainly affect how you show up.

Remember These

- The better you are offline, the better you'll look online.
- Your personal brand elicits conscious and subconscious reactions from anyone who meets, talks to, or hears about you.
- Conduct yourself *as if* you're already filling the job of your dreams.
- Keep your offline and online personas consistent with each other.
- When you're authentic, you're aware of your abilities and accomplishments but at the same time humbled by your own limitations, weaknesses, and work-in-progress status. This kind of authenticity is important to your brand because it makes you relatable.
- Err on the side of caution and agonize too much, rather than too little, over an online post instead of letting

$\longrightarrow$

everything fly without considering the consequences. When in doubt, don't.

- You have only a few seconds to make as strong a first impression as possible and to judge or make up your mind about those who are standing in front of you.

- How much or how little of your personality to take with you to the workplace is up to you. But be aware that, in the professional setting, you must make sure your personal brand sends the message you want to convey. The same is expected of you on social media.

- Just like networking in person, networking online isn't about meeting someone and immediately asking for the "sale." It's about getting to know people and building relationships—relationships that can provide mutual benefits for months and years down the road.

REFERENCE

Gladwell, M. 2007. *Blink: The Power of Thinking Without Thinking*. New York: Back Bay Books.

CHAPTER 7

Identify and Develop Your Leadership Style

Our emerging workforce is not interested in command-and-control leadership. They don't want to do things because I said so; they want to do things because they want to do them.

—*Irene Rosenfeld, former CEO, Mondelēz International*

Reading Points

- Follow
- Learn from Mistakes
- Show You Care
- Pay Attention to Culture
- Take Ownership
- Be Cognizant of the Company You Keep
- Build on Your Inherent Strengths and Talents

DON'T WAIT UNTIL you're a CEO, director, vice president, or some other high-level executive to start adopting approaches that enhance your leadership style and performance. By then, it will be too late. You'll have already etched in people's minds your personal brand that follows you from one organization to the next. And people's long-held perceptions are the hardest to convert. So start now, when you've just entered the healthcare door. You don't have to be a formal leader to act like a leader.

This chapter highlights good practices that any professional at any level can adopt to boost interaction, work performance, influence, and effect on others. We present them in no particular order because, at the end of the day, only you can decide which approach should take precedence over another.

FOLLOW

Followers get a bad rap in our individualistic society. Parents scold their children with the classic don't-be-a-follower line, "If all your friends jumped off a bridge, would you jump, too?!" Adults label those who conform as *sheeple*. *Hanger-on, peon, yes-man, minion,* and many other unflattering terms are indiscriminately used to describe a person who proudly supports or serves another. Hollywood perpetuates the image of followers as boring and traditional and nonfollowers as romantic and modern.

But perception often skews the truth. And the truth is, not everyone can be a leader. The other truth is, being a follower is not the weak-willed obedience to a mindless activity, person, viewpoint, or rule that society wants us to believe it is—at least not in the workplace. Instead, being a follower is an act of active participation, especially if you're working for a participative leader. That is, if you choose to follow deliberately (not out of impulse, thrill, or blind faith), you typically have

- a reason, a motivation, or an agenda;
- trust or confidence in the person (she's proven she knows what she's doing) or in the idea (everything will work out as planned);

- a desire to contribute something (including moral support) that helps the person or activity to function or move forward;
- team or group orientation (you believe you can accomplish more or achieve better results with others than on your own); and
- critical thinking skills that allow you to identify the pros and cons of what you're getting into.

Robert Kelley (1992), one of the first academics to examine the concept of followership in the workplace, estimated that followers "actually contribute more than 80 percent to the success of any project, any organization, while leaders at best contribute only 20 percent." Think about that. It means two things: (1) Followers carry out the vision, strategies, and plans leaders have crafted; and (2) leaders use followers' feedback, recommendations, perspectives, opinions, observations, and so on to spark or polish their own ideas.

We think that what leaders (regardless of style) want, though, are more than just warm-bodied followers. They want *good* followers. And by that we mean those who not only possess the requisite competency, work ethic, and interpersonal skills but also

- are honest, trustworthy, credible, and respectful;
- don't take or give abuse;
- have problem-solving and creative skills;
- take full responsibility for their mistakes and take the initiative to correct them;
- are eager to learn and teach others;
- can and want to work with other people; and
- are not afraid of constructive feedback.

Followers of this caliber are self-starters and self-managers. They are role models for the rest of the team and may be called upon to run a meeting, monitor an initiative, or do other high-level tasks in the absence of the leader.

One of the often-repeated maxims of management is that to be good leaders, people must first learn to be good followers. Why? Because followership requires humility, listening more than talking, giving more than taking, learning more than teaching, and teaching more than dictating. Leadership should require the same. Following doesn't make a leader less decisive or less in control, but more secure in knowing that reliable and capable followers "have his back" and have the organization's best interest at heart.

Incorporate followership into your style and then watch yourself improve, little by little, at being a leader.

LEARN FROM MISTAKES

Errors, missteps, unfortunate circumstances, and bumps in the road are inevitable. They will happen during your career—several times. And *when* (never *if*) they do, they will hurt and cause you to become discouraged, wrestle with your identity, and lose your self-confidence. It's tempting to sulk, hide, make excuses, or blame someone else. But none of these reactions leads you to a workable solution. So brush off these negative thoughts and keep on truckin'! Don't let the mistakes damage you (your brand or your team) and make you ineffective. Instead, rise above them and listen to what they're telling you.

Mistakes typically sound the alarm on things that are being ignored, that need fixing or correcting, or that operate under false assumptions. Identify and then address those issues. Be honest with yourself. Ask for feedback and be receptive to criticisms. Consult with your support system or network (including your mentor). Apologize or express your regret.

If learning from your mistakes is good, learning from others' mistakes is even better. Your mentor, coworkers, boss, CEO and other executives in your organization, and associates in your network are fantastic sources in this regard. Ask them (if you've already established a rapport) what their most embarrassing mistake has been so far and what they learned from it. Observe, if you can, how they handle mistakes. You won't know all the details, but you'll have a general idea of the what, the how, and the why. Add this information to your understanding and experience. You never know, one day you could apply these secondhand lessons to your own challenges.

SHOW YOU CARE

Allow others to see that you care. Don't do a kind thing once in a while just to show off to people that you're "caring," like the jerk who brings donuts on Fridays but routinely treats support staff like dirt all week long. People—from the CEO to the receptionist—will see right through you! Be authentic. Show others that your healthcare career is not just a job but a true calling, a passion. Show others that you're there to serve.

So how should you show (not just say) that you care? Here are a few suggestions.

1. *Treat everyone with respect and kindness*—every day, no matter what mood you're in, and despite whatever pressures you're facing. Don't do it to be magnanimous or to impress an audience. Do it because you're a decent human being.

2. *Learn and fully participate in the culture.* "When in Rome, do as the Romans do," as the adage goes. For you, it means embracing the unofficial and staff-driven rules, traditions,

and mores of your department and the organization. Don't criticize or make fun of the culture, and if you find something inappropriate or uncomfortable about it, let it go or talk to your boss. If you can't participate, do so without making a fuss.

3. *Do the right thing.* This may be easier said than done because in healthcare it isn't always easy to tell the "good" from the "bad" side, especially during a conflict. But do weigh both sides or the pros and cons of each. Lean on your convictions. Follow policies. Seek advice from others in the organization. Communicate with the parties involved. Being thoughtful about how you approach a problem sends a message that you are doing your best to make things right.

4. *Show up—and be prepared and on time.* When you show up ready, things get done. And when things get done, people see that you are there to work as hard as they do, that you care about their time and don't want to waste it, and that you're trying hard to do your part.

5. *Offer help and moral support.* This is a small gesture that means a lot. It builds people's morale, lets them know they are not alone, and relieves some of their stress.

Other ways you can show you care include being sympathetic and empathetic, acknowledging people's contributions and accomplishments, joining in on the fun (whether it's a potluck or a small birthday party or a company picnic), and not being a pushover or not making the tough but appropriate and fair call. (Allowing people to take advantage of your kindness is not a way to show you care.)

Having a caring and authentic leadership style encourages those around you to be less defensive and to up their game to match yours. Over time, your efforts to show you care compound and your influence on others grows.

PAY ATTENTION TO CULTURE

The way we do things around here. That's the most direct way of defining organizational culture, which exists in every company and even in departments. The culture could be as eccentric as an older gentleman standing in the lobby to greet passersby and urge them to play the piano nearby. Or as amazing as an ongoing competition over which nurses' station can drink the most office coffee every month. Or as endearing as an annual clown parade thrown by a children's hospital for its patients and their parents but attended by the entire community.

When you become part of a culture, don't be just a spectator, laughing and clapping on the sidelines. You gotta get in it! Play the piano even if you don't know how. Join the nurses for a cup o' joe. Offer to hand out candy during the parade.

When Natalie began her first CEO position at a small critical access hospital in Colorado, she wanted to immediately immerse herself in the community's culture. She was set on proving that she was happy to be there and eager to get to know the people. So what did she do? Within the first six months, she enrolled in night school and earned an EMT certificate to serve the town's voluntary ambulance department, graduated from square dancing lessons, went combining for corn with the chairman of the hospital's board of directors, learned to shoot clay pigeons, and joined the local gun club. She left all her dark business suits in her closet and embraced the adventure.

Natalie took the same approach in the hospital. Through close observation, she discovered that the cook, who had worked there for decades, was one of the most beloved employees. Everyone valued and respected her opinion. As such, she represented the informal leaders in the organization. Natalie knew that if she wanted to understand the culture, she could question the cook and learn.

Informal leaders are important because they have a strong influence on other staff. Getting to know them is like getting a taste or a whiff of what's cooking in the organization, so to speak. Informal leaders know or represent how the rest of the employees think, how they may react to a change initiative, what they may find acceptable and nonnegotiable, and what they may support or push back against.

If your leadership style is strategic, make a habit of being involved in the culture, including the subcultures. Identify how the leader's style makes or breaks a culture and inspires the best performance.

TAKE OWNERSHIP

Cerner Corporation, a healthcare software company based in Kansas City, Missouri, teaches every new employee the company principle called "kill the snake" (Sorensen 2014). No, the company's staff aren't reptile haters. The phrase means if you see a problem, fix it. Doesn't matter whose problem. Doesn't matter who caused it. You spotted it, you take care of it. Period. Cerner warns its employees never to see a snake and then walk away from it as if it didn't rear its ugly head. That snake will one day come back and bite everyone.

This philosophy perfectly exemplifies what taking ownership is all about. It's not about taking the fall for someone else; it's about looking out for the interest of the whole group, not just your own, so that no one takes a tumble—but if that happens, that person is not going to fall alone. In other words, taking ownership is a *we* thing, not an *I* thing.

When you take ownership of a project, for example, you are fully engaged. You care that everyone involved is doing their part according to the time line, the objectives, the expected quality, and so on. If they are not, then you offer help for the sake of moving the project forward. If the project turns out to be unsatisfactory, you share the blame and the responsibility for fixing the issue—even though you did your part correctly. If the project turns out well, you congratulate everyone for a job well done and share the credit.

While you work, do you kill the snake? If not, how do you handle that snake when it reappears? Do you do a lot of work-arounds or engage in redundancies because of it? How can you adjust your style to take ownership of problems and do your job more efficiently?

BE COGNIZANT OF THE COMPANY YOU KEEP

Think about your immediate family, then your extended family. Think about your significant other, close friends, and acquaintances. Think about your mentors and advisors. Think about your coworkers, including your boss and everyone else you work with. Think about your social media network or followers. All these people are in your sphere of influence—the people you have influence over and who have influence over you. These people shape who you are personally and professionally and are part of the reasons you do what you do. Now, answer these questions:

- Who pushes you to be a better person?
- Who encourages you in all your pursuits, including personal and professional development?
- Who gave you the idea to go into healthcare management?
- Who are your biggest influencers?
- Who is just like you—same profession, same ambition, same short-term and long-term goals, same attitude, and so on?
- Who helps you set goals and change habits?
- Who is most and least responsive to you—either online or offline?
- Who is your cheerleader?
- Who is your rock?

- Who can you always turn to for help, to talk to, or to confide in?
- Who is your biggest critic (outside of you)? Naysayer? Rival?
- Who discourages or makes fun of your personal and professional efforts?
- Whose life, career path, future goals, and general beliefs used to mimic yours but are now opposite from yours?
- Do you consider the people who surround you a negative or a positive force in your life?
- Who affects you positively or negatively? In what way?
- Do you like hanging out with them? If not, why not?
- Are you outgrowing some of your friends? Are they outgrowing you? Do you still share something in common with them? If not, why not?
- Whom haven't you seen or talked to in at least one year?
- Whom do you need or want to cut ties with?

Asking yourself these questions reveals who in your sphere of influence affects you the most and the least, and what effect those people have on you. Negative influencers can push you off course and leave you stranded, while positive influencers will pull you in the right direction. By occasionally taking this inventory, you can decide to decrease or increase the amount of time you spend with certain people. You may find that you've outgrown some people or that your views and priorities are no longer in sync with theirs. (Exhibit 7.1 discusses two theories of influence.)

The company you keep has the power to strengthen or weaken your performance. If your sphere of influence is supportive and enthusiastic about your efforts to grow personally and professionally, then chances are you will stay committed and disciplined. If your sphere of influence is discouraging or lacks interest in what you're doing, then you could lose your focus and churn out mediocre work.

Exhibit 7.1 The Average Five and the Sixth Man Theories

Motivational speaker Jim Rohn (2012) theorizes that "you are the average of the five people closest to you." That means almost everything an adult is—character, behavior, abilities, fears, occupation or ambition, accomplishments, failures, likes and dislikes, and so on—is shaped or influenced by the people she spends the most time with. And she, in turn, influences someone else's life, and on it goes. As a result, each of us has beliefs and interests that mirror those of our friends, family members, and significant others.

For example, if you're a fitness freak, your best friend is too. If you're religious or political or into social activism, one or both of your parents may have passed that value on to you. And if you're a spendthrift or extravagant, you learned that behavior from someone close to you now or in the past.

The lesson is simple: Be mindful and deliberate about selecting people to associate with. Befriend those whose interests are similar or complementary to yours or from whom you can learn a lot. Let go of those whose presence or influence is negative.

Apply this theory to yourself. Does it work for you?

Now let's extend this concept to what we'll call "the sixth man" (patterned after the Texas A&M football program's twelfth man notion of its fans being the twelfth member of the 11-man team on the field). The sixth man doesn't have to be a man or even a person. It's a force that represents the thing (not person) that causes you to do what you do. It could be your spirit, free will, words of wisdom or words of doubt, a hole inside you that needs to be filled, that thing that keeps you up at night, a goal or dream, a hobby, and so on. Let's give an example.

Many years ago, we both had the privilege of meeting the brilliant Ben Carson, secretary of the Department of Housing and Urban Development and retired pediatric neurosurgeon. He grew up dirt-poor in Detroit. His mother worked as a housekeeper for wealthy families and noticed that their homes had shelves and shelves stuffed with books. She realized then that these financially successful families had something in common: They all read. Although she couldn't read, she decided to instill a love of books in her children by simply encouraging them to read every day. Reading and learning gave each of her children the drive to succeed, and all of them turned out to be highly accomplished. That encouragement to

(continued)

read was Carson's sixth man. He has received many merit awards for his work and contributions to the scientific and medical fields, among them the highest civilian award in the United States—the Presidential Medal of Freedom.

All influences are valid, but the sixth man is the kind that doesn't quit provoking you until you do something about it. Be aware of your environment. Are you observant and learning from it, or drifting aimlessly through life, not gleaning insight from the journey?

BUILD ON YOUR INHERENT STRENGTHS AND TALENTS

Take a blank piece of paper and draw a vertical line down the center to make two columns. In one column, sign your name as many times as possible using your dominant hand. In the other column, do the same thing but with your nondominant hand.

Unless you are truly ambidextrous, the two columns will look vastly different. One side is legible, while the other resembles a four-year-old's scribbling. How did it feel signing with your nondominant hand? Frustrating? Awkward? Tedious? Slow?

This feeling perfectly demonstrates the struggle of developing weaknesses rather than honing innate strengths. We're not saying you shouldn't improve weaknesses—by all means, do! In fact, the premise of this book is development. But building up the talents or inclinations that you already possess and that engage you should not take a back seat, either, because strengths-based improvement delivers a more engaging and sustainable reward.

For example, consider a young, introverted chief financial officer. She prefers to work independently so she can focus on her tasks. But her boss, the autocratic system CEO, wants her to start presenting financial reports twice a year to the system and hospital boards. And pronto! He doesn't give her enough time to prepare or consider her ability to present. She is panicked because she hates public speaking and collaborating with other departments and staffs. Her new responsibility means she has to take public speaking classes and then prepare slides and practice before each presentation—on top of performing all her other duties. Normally, she's confident, highly competent, and a finance wizard. During her presentations, though, she sweats and stutters and second-guesses herself when she is asked a question. Because of all the time she spends on her presentations, her regular job begins to suffer. After just three presentations, she quits her job.

That's a total waste of talent!

Before you can hone your strengths, you must accurately identify them. How do you do that? Here are some simple, straightforward methods:

1. Ask for feedback from your sphere of influence and other trusted sources.

2. Look through past performance reviews and focus on areas in which you excelled.

3. Observe yourself at work for at least one week and take notes. What gets you excited? What grabs your attention or piques your interest? What do you find most rewarding? What puts you in a steady state of "don't bother me, I'm doing something"?

4. Take an aptitude or competency test. One powerful tool is StrengthsFinder. Don Clifton—founder of the Clifton StrengthsFinder, Gallup's online psychological assessment—is known as the father of the strengths-based movement. The catalyst of this movement was a 1950s research study on a speed-reading course. The study found that the greatest growth in ability occurred among students who were already reading at an above-average rate of speed. The average readers started at 90 words per minute (wpm) and the speed-reading course improved their speed to 150 wpm, an increase of 67 percent. The above-average readers, on the other hand, started at 350 wpm and went up to 2,900 wpm, an improvement of about 800 percent!

    The StrengthsFinder tool is based on the idea that you have the most opportunity to improve in areas in which you are already strong. For example, if you're highly analytical, you have a better chance of deepening that expertise than someone who has average analytical abilities. Similarly, if you're a natural people person, you're better at building and strengthening relationships and connections than someone who is independent. Find the StrengthsFinder tool at www.strengthsfinder.com/home.aspx. For another method, see exhibit 7.2.

The more you refine your talents and focus on the things you do well (instead of poorly), the more confident you become and the better your overall performance gets (even in areas that don't come naturally to you). The reverse is also true: The more you beat yourself up over your weaknesses and your deficiencies, the lower your self-esteem gets and the more mistakes you commit.

Exhibit 7.2 Better Than 10,000 Others

What do you do better than 10,000 others? This is a question Laurie often poses during her consulting sessions. The typical first response is, "Are you kidding?! I have nothing that special to offer." But with a little prodding, attendees begin to share with their small groups. And then something beautiful happens. The room comes alive with the din of chatter and exchange of ideas. Instead of individuals talking about their personal strengths, group members heap praises on each other:

- Donna is such a deep well of knowledge. Every time I have a complex patient case, I always consult her.

- Robin is so beloved by our patients. The first question out of their mouths is, "Where's Robin?"

- Erika is so good at solving problems. When the network server crashes or the electronic health record software is not responding, she can troubleshoot and get us right back on track.

Do you know why it's so hard for people to answer this question? Often, we hear only the complaints about our performance or an exhortation to work on our weak areas. We seldom hear praise for what we did right. Is it any wonder, then, that people don't think they outperform even two other people, let alone 10,000?

> ### *Remember These*
>
> - Being a follower is an act of active participation.
> - Followers "actually contribute more than 80 percent to the success of any project, any organization, while leaders at best contribute only 20 percent."
> - Culture can be defined as "the way we do things around here."
> - "Kill the snake" means if you see a problem, fix it. It's about taking ownership.
> - The company you keep has the power to strengthen or weaken your performance. If your sphere of influence is supportive and enthusiastic about your efforts to grow personally and professionally, then chances are you will stay committed and disciplined. If your sphere of influence is discouraging or lacks interest in what you're doing, then you could lose your focus and churn out mediocre work.
> - Building up the talents that you already possess and that engage you should not take a back seat to improving your weaknesses because strengths-based improvement delivers a more engaging and sustainable reward.

REFERENCES

Kelley, R. E. 1992. *The Power of Followership: How to Create Leaders People Want to Follow and Followers Who Lead Themselves.* New York: Doubleday.

Rohn, J. 2012. *My Philosophy for Successful Living.* Melrose, FL: No Dream Too Big LLC.

Sorensen, A. 2014. Personal communication with the authors, April.

ADDITIONAL RESOURCES

Atchison, T. A. 2003. *Followership: A Practical Guide to Aligning Leaders and Followers.* Chicago: Health Administration Press.

Bass, B. M., and R. E. Riggio. 2008. *Transformational Leadership*. Mahwah, NJ: Lawrence Erlbaum Associates.

Kelley, R. E. 1988. "In Praise of Followers." *Harvard Business Review*. Published November. http://hbr.org/1988/11/in-praise-of-followers/ar/1.

Rath, T. 2007. *StrengthsFinder 2.0*. Lincoln, NE: Gallup Press.

Rath, T., and B. Conchie. 2009. *Strengths-Based Leadership 2.0*. Lincoln, NE: Gallup Press.

Note to My 25-Year-Old Self

As I turned 25, I was graduating from medical school in Brooklyn, New York, after a challenging and transformational four years. If I knew then what I know now, here is what I would write to my 25-year-old self.

Dear Frank:

You've just come through a difficult period. Congratulations! You've made mistakes and sacrifices, achieved success, and endured failure, but you're still in the game. I would like to provide a few words of advice.

1. *Always remember that it's not about you.* You have been given a wonderful opportunity for one reason: to help others. If you focus your efforts on serving others and meeting their needs, it will work out for you—better than you could ever imagine. Those who focus solely on their own self-interest are generally not successful and usually unhappy.

2. *Be less patient with systems and more patient with people, including yourself.* Sometimes it will seem that every issue, large or small, real or imagined, is a "hair on fire" crisis. That approach will be exhausting, distracting, and unhealthy, both for you and for those around you. Fortunately, the intensive care unit nurses you work with will tell you, "We can do this the easy way, or we can do this the hard way," and they will assure you (correctly) that you wouldn't like the hard way. They will teach you about team care before it becomes a cliché and give you an awesome gift. You won't have to pretend you have the answer key—you won't. You can say, "I don't know, what do you think?" to your colleagues and solve problems as a team, to benefit the patients you are privileged to serve together. This will be helpful in both your clinical and administrative roles.

3. *Work hard but take care of yourself—your job doesn't love you back.* The primary filter in your career decision-making

algorithm must be what is best for your family, you, and your career. It is not selfish to seek meaningful work where you can make a difference, in an organization whose values and goals are aligned with your personal hopes and dreams. Organizations change, values change, leaders change, and the type of leadership needed changes. Work hard every day, and when you leave an organization you will owe, and be owed, nothing. Leave organizations on positive terms, because the road runs in both directions. And you will finally learn to take better care of yourself after you develop an ulcer in your third year of practice.

4. *Manage transitions well.* Life is managing a series of transitions because change is life's only constant. The day you start your pulmonary medicine fellowship, your mentor and role model will announce he is leaving. Rather than despairing, you will carefully select another great mentor. Later, you will realize you can make more of a difference by switching from clinical medicine to administrative medicine. And you will find even more fulfillment bringing the clinical perspective into the boardroom and administrative suite, reaching decisions by asking, "What will this mean to those who are receiving and providing care?"

5. *Pay attention to the duties you don't like to do.* Every job is a Venn diagram with two circles: the tasks you like to do and those you have to do. You will be fortunate because those circles will overlap a lot; however, they will not be concentric. Identify the job duties you dislike and do them well. Leaders who ignore the things they don't like do so at their own peril.

6. *Nurture relationships.* When your mentor, Dave Ridderheim, LFACHE, hires you for your first full-time administrative role, you will think he spends too much time on relationships. Fortunately, you will quickly realize he had it just right. The trusting, collaborative relationships he developed are the bedrock on which Parkview Health will be built during a wave of rapid consolidation in the mid-1990s. Focus on building relationships for the long term, not simply to consummate an immediate transaction. Also, the future is multidisciplinary and interdisciplinary. Build relationships with people outside your discipline and in other groups, professions, and organizations

throughout your community. To serve your community, you must know your community. That won't happen if you just sit in your office. Spend time with people who are different from you, personally and professionally. You will build some of your more fulfilling and enduring relationships this way.

7. *You must be present to win.* Leave it all on the field every day. Engage with your patients and your colleagues. Improve your listening skills, in both your personal and professional life.

8. *Learn how to say no.* Your wife Cindy will say, "It's exhausting being around you!" Your reply, "It's exhausting being me! And saying yes is a lot more fun than saying no," is not the correct one. To contribute your best to the most critical priorities, both personally and professionally, be disciplined and choose wisely where you invest your time and talent.

9. *Don't sell your musical equipment to pay your college tuition.* Although you will later acquire new instruments and music will again become an important part of your life, allowing you to play in bands for more than 30 years, you will always regret the nine-year gap. And you won't be very knowledgeable about the music of the late 1970s and early 1980s. Personal hobbies and passions allow driven professionals to find a creative outlet and strike balance in busy lives.

10. *Spoiler alert: It will all work out.* You will enjoy learning the stories of people you meet, as they share the twists and turns of life. You'll have fun thinking about the massive odds against everyone present being in the same room, given the different life paths taken. When people share their inspiring story of the obstacles they've overcome and the challenges they've faced, they usually conclude, "But it all worked out." You will tell them, "It all worked out because you made it work out. It worked out because you refused to let it not work out. It worked out because you didn't curl up in the fetal position when the going got tough!" That will be your story, too.

Signed,
Frank D. Byrne, MD, FACHE, FACPE, FACP, FCCP
President Emeritus, SSM Health St. Mary's Hospital
Senior Executive Advisor, HealthX Ventures

CHAPTER 8

Try, or Find Inspiration in, Servant Leadership

Good leaders must first become good servants.

—Robert K. Greenleaf, founder, Greenleaf Center
for Servant Leadership

Reading Points

- The Benefits of Servant Leadership

- The Unassuming Acts of Servant Leaders

- Choosing to Be Brave, Not Popular

- Joining or Starting Difficult Conversations

WHAT KIND OF leader do you want to be? There are many leadership styles to choose from. But if you want to be a leader who has a reputation for putting other people first, then it's time you look into servant leadership.

Servant leadership might as well be called *selfless leadership*. Because it isn't about you. It's about your audience, your stakeholders, your constituents (yep, like a politician; did you know every healthcare leader has a dual role as a politician?). These constituents include the organization's senior leaders, board of directors, management, employees (including your staff, if you have them), patients and their families, physicians, and community members and business leaders. Servant leadership is only about you in the sense that you are the one doing the serving. You have to commit to serving the needs and wants of others to help them become extraordinary.

Like everything else in the book, becoming a servant leader takes years, which is likely why this style is mostly associated with senior leaders. But you can begin this journey now. There is enormous value in serving your stakeholders in the early years of your career.

So how can you get started?

First, practice the strategies we offer in this and other chapters. We say this not to give lip service to our own recommendations but to drive home the point that many of the concepts we discuss—self-awareness, humility, emotional intelligence, personal growth or learning, commitment and self-discipline, followership, integrity, and building trust and relationships—share the same philosophy with servant leadership. Each of these strategies will get you closer to becoming a servant leader.

Second, be kind—or at the very least, be nice. Simple as that. You don't have to be a saint, but you do have to be considerate, courteous, helpful, and modest with everyone you deal with. Keep in mind that hiring managers also look for this character trait. They don't want to recruit and select job candidates who don't care, are arrogant, are selfish, or are rude. After all, it is much easier to teach skills to kind people than to teach kindness to skilled but mean people.

In this chapter, we continue to share improvement techniques we've learned from our more-than-15-years' experience in healthcare. But this time, we've set our eyes on practices that are intended to bring out the servant leader in you.

THE BENEFITS OF SERVANT LEADERSHIP

Let's clarify one concept: True servant leaders have altruistic intentions. They are servants not because they get money, power, prestige, or any other perks from it. They are servants because they see serving as a critical duty or responsibility (Greenleaf 1977). They provide encouragement, approval, resources, information, other necessary support, and even tough love so employees can do their jobs and do them well, and so the community or society can benefit.

This doesn't mean servant leadership offers no benefits for the person. One benefit is genuine influence, the kind that inspires (*not* requires) others to follow your vision, to be loyal to you, to perform their best work, and to become servant leaders themselves. You can't buy, take, or beg for that kind of influence. You have to earn it. Never assume that having a title (e.g., CEO, chief operating officer [COO], executive vice president, chief financial officer [CFO]) automatically means having genuine influence. No matter where you are in the organizational chart, influence is golden. But it's invaluable as your career progresses and when you reach the executive level because that's when more complicated decisions that require more stakeholder buy-in are made.

Another benefit of servant leadership is an enhanced reputation. Reputation is what other people think of you. You have no direct control over it. What you can control is your own behavior. If you act selflessly—for example, being a team player, volunteering to help, and supporting others' work and goals—people will notice. When you take such actions, their opinion of you improves, their trust and respect for you grows, and your credibility strengthens. Then, these same people will spread the word, guaranteeing that your reputation precedes you wherever you go. Of course, if you behave selfishly, word will spread faster—but not in a good way.

We've said this before, and we'll say it again: The little acts you commit every day matter, and they compound over time to create a big change or outcome. If you adopt servant leadership now—when the stakes are lower than if you're a titled executive—in a few years (perhaps even months) you will see that your influence has grown exponentially among those you serve day in and day out. Even if you change jobs or move on to another organization later in your career, your learned habit of serving others will be beneficial in so many ways.

THE UNASSUMING ACTS OF SERVANT LEADERS

Exercise these servant leader acts until they turn into habits.

Never Ask Someone Else to Do Something That You Couldn't or Wouldn't Do

Intimidated to approach the CFO about a complicated budget question or an overdue report? Don't send a team member on your behalf. Won't lie or cover up for anyone's mistake? Don't even insinuate to anyone to do the same for you when you mess up. Nothing says selfish or self-serving more than refusing to do or face a difficult, awkward, or potentially risky task and pushing it onto somebody else. That's cowardice and abuse of power, which people don't easily forget or forgive.

Another way of exercising this tiny act is to always be willing to roll up your sleeves and pitch in when needed. Servant leaders never think they are too high on the totem pole or too successful to do menial tasks or manual labor. They don't assign those tasks to their direct reports, and they are not content with just supervising the work; instead, they get involved and are happy for the opportunity to literally (not figuratively) get their hands dirty. Boxing emergency packages for the community after a natural disaster, answering phones on the patient care floor during a staff shortage or an unusually high patient census, and offering your expertise to help solve or prevent a problem are just some ways you can show you are not above doing things outside your official duties.

Say Yes to Every Opportunity to Help or Participate

By doing so, you are exposing yourself to new experiences and possibilities; learning about different roles, departments, settings, and processes; and meeting leaders and staff you would not encounter otherwise. Most important, you are creating goodwill between you and those you're serving. Immerse yourself in these experiences and absorb as many of their lessons as possible. Even (and especially) if an initiative or project doesn't turn out as planned, you can learn something that you can apply later.

Communicate Clearly and Regularly

Whether you're leading a big project team, supervising a small staff, or just going about your daily tasks, direct and regular communication is a service you're performing. How? When you speak clearly (and listen!), give simple instructions, define roles and expectations, share relevant information, provide and request updates, or check on progress and problems, you are empowering all involved in the project or in the exchange—whether staff members, bosses, doctors, or vendors and consultants—to do their part. Your communication is a guide, something for them to work with and work toward. Without communication, the work stalls, misunderstandings multiply, mistakes are made and not fixed, deadlines are ignored, and people get very angry. Plus, when you communicate, you're showing that you care and that you're there when people need you.

Don't Be Afraid to Ask the Question

Six little words can have a huge impact on your reputation or others' opinion of you. And no, they aren't *May I have a pay raise?* Those words are *Can you help me to understand?* Admitting you don't understand something is hard. But in showing that you don't know and that you need help, you gain not only the knowledge you need but also strong allies.

Don't underestimate the power of humility and vulnerability. When you admit that you don't fully understand something, the barriers between employees (no matter their titles) immediately disintegrate. There is no faster way to start a completely neutral, healthy, and productive discussion—and to move the conversation forward—than posing this question. Plus, it allows others to be of service to you. Who among us doesn't enjoy using our know-how to come to someone's aid? Who isn't flattered when asked to lend our expertise? This is especially true of healthcare professionals, who have built our lives around serving others.

Take this story as an example:

A hospital COO we know has made asking this question a habit. His background is nontraditional: He earned his stripes in the marketing and strategic planning realm of healthcare. He had limited exposure to the operational and clinical sides. Because of this background, others were often quick to dismiss him, unsure of his credibility. At first, he reacted by being defensive. He even doubted his own abilities. But then he developed a better approach. He began to ask, "Can you help me to understand?" It was such a simple request, but it disarmed those he was talking to and led them to serve, teach, and collaborate rather than doubt and attack. He genuinely won them over.

Is the question scary? You bet! Worth it? Oh yeah.

CHOOSING TO BE BRAVE, NOT POPULAR

We all want to be liked. It's human nature. At work, you may be tempted to make everyone happy so that you will be liked. The danger of caving in to this temptation is that you may soften the blow of bad news, fail to set performance expectations for your employees or team members, share information that is not intended for disclosure, or turn a blind eye to bad behavior or abuses of power (especially by your work friends). These acts are directly opposite those practiced by servant leaders, who are experts at building relationships but savvy about not crossing boundaries.

Did you know that what gets you liked in the long run often involves making unpopular, nerve-racking decisions in the short run? Focus on that long game. That's where the payoff is. Don't let a self-centered desire to be liked drive your professional decisions. If the motivation for your decisions is simply to "make nice"—not because you have the best interests of the organization, its employees, and the community at heart—then you're doing everyone (including you) a disservice. Sure, you won't rock the boat this way, but you will certainly undermine your authority (not to mention your career down the road).

Instead of being liked, work toward being respected. Respect is equity that you earn through good behavior, service, hard work, and accomplishment. You could easily lose that equity, however. For example, discretion is crucial in leadership, and a breach of that discretion leads to loss of respect. If you share confidential or inside information to endear someone to you, that individual will see you as a person who cannot be trusted, not as a person who is open and honest. Any respect you've earned from that person will vanish.

Hold Others to High Standards

Having earned a Division I athletic scholarship, Natalie was sure she was ready for college-level track practice. Then she met her coach, a hard-driving but highly respected leader. His team's respect for him ran so deep that all members pushed themselves beyond their personal limits to win meets and perform at their best. During his rigorous practices, Natalie would run off the track to throw up from exhaustion. She would quickly compose herself and then return to finish her workout. That happened a few times, especially in her first semester of college. The coach (and his assistants) didn't tolerate excuses or complaints, nor did he care whether the team liked his decisions. He knew what every athlete on his team was capable of, and he held each of them to very high standards. Despite his toughness, everyone clearly understood that he was coming from a good place: He only wanted what was best for the team and the individual athletes; he wasn't doing it for his own good. Natalie pushed through the long, grueling practices and became efficient at writing term papers on the long bus rides to and from meets. Her self-discipline, tenacity, and time management skills—not to mention her physical fitness and running times—only improved because of this experience. All thanks to a brave coach who wasn't afraid to make the unpopular decisions that serve the interests of his athletes.

Laurie's science teacher in high school also was demanding. She wasn't adored by her students, and her teaching style was an acquired taste. She refused to let anyone slack off. But she knew science and was adamant that every student learn it. What Laurie didn't realize until many years later was that this teacher wasn't tough because she was mean-spirited. In fact, quite the opposite: She was difficult because she cared a lot about the students' future. She pushed them to turn in their best work and to think critically. She drilled into them not just scientific principles but also discipline and structure. These principles contributed to Laurie's growth and stay with her today.

Like the coach and the science teacher, you should hold your constituents (not to mention yourself) to a higher standard. It's not easy to do; you certainly will not win any popularity contests and you may feel left out. But as a future leader, you have to start making the tough calls for the benefit of the people you serve (not just for your benefit). That will earn you respect, which is much more valuable than being liked. We're not asking you to be icy or hostile; in fact, we encourage you to be warm and caring. What we're asking you to be is courageous—to do the right things for the greatest number of people.

JOINING OR STARTING DIFFICULT CONVERSATIONS

"If you're not at the table, you can bet you're on the menu." Have you heard that saying? It's silly, but it makes a great point. If you don't start or join the difficult conversation, you will be counted out.

When (never *if*) you fail or make a mistake, the next steps should include a discussion about what went wrong, what you did and didn't do, and how you can prevent the mistake next time. This conversation is difficult and awkward, and you might delay, avoid, or skip it. And we can't blame you; we know what that's like. (See chapter 9 for more discussion on failure.)

But if you keep stalling this conversation, what would your constituents say about you? Would they start to doubt your ability to lead and serve them? Postponing it doesn't make the issues disappear. In fact, they undoubtedly will only get worse.

What do you think would happen if you do sit down at the table? You may get an earful, sure. But criticism to your face is always better than criticism behind your back. Be prepared to approach the meeting with humility, and answer questions, apologize, take ownership, and offer solutions. The conversation will end soon enough, and you'll feel relieved and proud for having faced the music once and for all. Plus, you'll come away with some lessons learned, and you'll certainly earn the respect of your team, staff, and even boss just for showing up.

Joining or starting difficult conversations (whether related to failures or something else) is a test of your commitment to serve. If you step up, you've passed. You're sending a message to others that, despite your fears of confrontations and despite setbacks, you're there to continue your service and there when you're needed most.

Servant leaders don't quit when the going gets tough. Neither should you.

Remember These

- Servant leadership isn't about you. It's about your audience, your stakeholders, your constituents.

- Becoming a servant leader takes years, which is likely why this style is mostly associated with senior leaders. But you can begin this journey now. There is enormous value in serving your stakeholders in the early years of your career.

- Many of the concepts we discuss—self-awareness, humility, emotional intelligence, personal growth or learning, commitment and self-discipline, followership, integrity, and building trust and relationships—share the same philosophy with servant leadership. Each of these strategies will get you closer to becoming a servant leader.

- Be nice. Simple as that. You don't have to be a saint, but you do have to be considerate, courteous, helpful, and modest with everyone you deal with. Keep in mind that hiring managers also look for this character trait.

- True servant leaders have altruistic intentions. They are servants not because they get money, power, prestige, or any other perks from it. They are servants because they see serving as a critical duty or responsibility.

- One benefit of being a servant leader is genuine influence, the kind that inspires (*not* requires) others to follow your vision, to be loyal to you, to perform their best work, and to become servant leaders themselves.

- Another benefit of servant leadership is an enhanced reputation. Reputation is what other people think of you. If you act selflessly—for example, being a team player, volunteering to help, and supporting others' work and goals—people will notice. That's when their opinion of you improves, their trust and respect for you grows, and your credibility strengthens.

REFERENCE

Greenleaf, R. 1977. *Servant Leadership*. Mahwah, NJ: Paulist Press.

Note to My 25-Year-Old Self

Looking back over my career, I reflect on the great privilege it has been to serve organizations that had a mission and values that were aligned with my personal mission and values. The opportunity to be part of a calling that is larger than me provides immeasurable enrichment. We in healthcare are particularly fortunate to serve others at their time of greatest need. Very early in my career, as an administrative resident, I had two mentors whose values were wholly focused on serving the patient and the greater good, using the organization's resources. The selfless example of others who went before me served to guide my own path. I advise emerging leaders today to seek to work for an organization whose mission and values are congruent with their own.

My words of wisdom to my 25-year-old self would be to *achieve more work–life balance*. Take time and be present with family and friends, and invest in self-renewal. This is challenging when serving a 24-7 mission. That being said, your organization will be better served when you are fully engaged at both home and work.

As you advance in your career, you will be called upon to make increasingly difficult decisions. Exercising good judgment requires sound values, solid preparation, and an effective and ready team. Your team may include employees, your board of directors or key advisors, and your family. Surround yourself with great people who will hold you accountable. Encourage others, and ask them to encourage you.

Lead by example. Seek to learn, grow, and succeed, but do so with mindfulness toward balance and prudence. This is a time of great change in our industry, compounded by rapidly increasing technology and accessibility. Leverage the technology available to you, but make time to unplug and recharge. If you're stressed out all the time, you'll make more mistakes and may not interact with your team as effectively as you could. As a leader, if you don't take time for yourself and your family and friends, it can send a message or expectation that others cannot take that needed time, either.

While planning your career and considering strategic transitions, seek wise counsel from advisors, colleagues, and mentors. Listen, consider, and then trust your instincts. In 1981, I was an associate administrator in a large hospital of a multihospital system. I was presented with an opportunity to become the CEO of a 60-bed rural hospital in the system. Most of my advisors felt that it would be a mistake, that I wouldn't advance from there. But it felt like the right choice, and I followed my gut. After one year (of having the best time of my career), I was reassigned—this time as CEO of a 400-bed community hospital in the system. I don't believe that would have happened if I hadn't demonstrated experience leading as CEO of a smaller facility. Ultimately, you have to do what you feel is best. You own your own career. Reflect; consider where you feel called, where you can best serve; and make a difference. I am grateful for the support of my family to make moves and transitions throughout my career. Don't look back and regret. Make courageous and strategic decisions.

Be yourself. Discover and understand your strengths and weaknesses. Surround yourself with people who buttress your limitations. Embrace diversity of thought, and be intentional to seek out those with contrasting experience, expertise, and perspective. Be transparent in your weaknesses, and empower others to contribute where you are less disposed. Your authenticity will engender the trust and confidence of those around you. Seek candid feedback on how you can improve as a leader, and set an example and expectation that others do the same.

Be engaged in your profession. Affiliation and involvement in the American College of Healthcare Executives (ACHE) has been invaluable in equipping me as a leader. ACHE offers tremendous professional education and development resources, publications, and tools that increase effectiveness. Its board certification process equips and validates your credibility. For me, however, the most powerful value of ACHE is the network of colleagues it offers. I've met people who have helped me develop my network, who have been my best and most candid advisors, and who were there when I have faced challenges. I heartily encourage you to engage and advance.

Signed,
William C. Schoenhard, LFACHE
Chairman (2006–2007), American College of Healthcare Executives
Former (Retired) Deputy Under Secretary for Health for Operations and Management, US Department of Veterans Affairs

CHAPTER 9

Bounce Back from Failure

Mistakes are the usual bridge between inexperience and wisdom.

—*Phyllis Theroux, essayist*

Reading Points

- Managing Failure
- Taking and Handling Criticism
- Persevering Through the Nos
- Trying New Things
- Forgetting

DID YOU KNOW?

- Michael Jordan was cut from his high school basketball team.
- Walt Disney was fired from a newspaper for "lacking imagination" and "having no original ideas."
- Steve Jobs was unceremoniously removed from the company he started.

- Oprah Winfrey was demoted from her job as a news anchor because she "wasn't fit for television."
- The Beatles were rejected by a recording studio, which said, "We don't like their sound, they have no future in show business."

This list could go on and on, but our point is this: Failures happen to everyone, even to very talented, famous people. As we've said, failures are a matter of *when*, never a matter of *if*. All we can do is hope for the best, but plan for the worst.

Don't define your career in this constantly changing, high-stress, high-stakes healthcare industry by the number of times you failed or made a mistake. Doing so is unfair, and it diminishes the countless things you've accomplished, contributed, and improved. Instead, see failure for what it is—an inevitable and scary occurrence that you can bounce back and learn from and you can prevent. How you overcome or rebound from adversity is what should define your career, because that's tough work that not only requires but also shows your strength of character—whether you're tenacious, resilient, committed, disciplined, progress oriented, and so on.

Many of us were schooled to believe that failure is bad. But that's only true if you let it stop you from trying again. In fact, failure is good because it provides learning and growth opportunities. It also promotes taking risks by applying new approaches to old or existing processes. The corporate giant 3M, for example, has a companywide philosophy that encourages employees to fail—and do so regularly (Kalb 2013). If employees aren't failing 95 percent of the time, the company reasons, then they likely aren't trying anything fresh and current. Although we elevate our chances of falling flat on our faces if the new techniques don't work, the fact that we ventured out to test new waters is valuable. It expands not only our skills but also our professional and personal horizons.

In this chapter, we challenge you to rethink your ideas about failure. We provide tips for managing failure, facing criticism and rising above it, and persevering despite rejections.

MANAGING FAILURE

Early careerists who are new to healthcare enjoy a grace period (although this varies from organization to organization) in which they are afforded some leeway to learn their roles and responsibilities and to adjust to the environment. This "honeymoon" period is a great time for you to establish good habits, including managing failure or what to do when you make a mistake.

During this time, when you are eager to pursue projects, participate in activities, and prove yourself, the likelihood that you will fail at least once is high. If it does happen, stay calm. It's not the end of the world. Handle the situation as graciously, humbly, and professionally as you can. The grace you show at this time will be noted by your colleagues, bosses, and even patients or their families. More important, it will set you up to successfully handle more complicated failures as your career progresses.

Here are our suggested ways to manage failure:

- *Admit your part in the failure.* Acknowledging your mistake, often publicly, is the only way you can begin to learn and to pick up the broken pieces and start over. An admission requires bravery and humility, as there may be a lot of criticisms of your actions and scrutiny of your work processes. Explain and share information, and listen more than talk.
- *Reject rejection.* As painful and disappointing as a failure is, it shouldn't have so much power that it paralyzes you emotionally and mentally. Don't allow that to happen. Dwell on the failure if you must, but don't dwell too long.

The more time you spend on beating yourself up, the less time you spend on recovering, learning, and moving on. Bounce back!

- *Put failure in perspective.* Failure is a temporary, isolated setback. Many (if not most) of the workplace mistakes you make are one-time events, not patterns. If resolved appropriately, they don't escalate or cause permanent damage. If you learned from them and committed to not repeating them, they don't recur. Have some perspective. If you see every failure as a career-ending, reputation-ruining event, you are only elevating your fear.

- *See failure as part of the success process.* There's no such thing as an overnight success. Even those who have won the lottery usually bought tickets for years before they hit the jackpot. When we landed our respective executive jobs at an early age, we had been paying dues formally and informally for several years to position ourselves for the next big thing. Success not only takes time but also involves failures—a lot of them. When you view failure as just another part of the success process, like acing a job interview and getting a promotion, then you're taking away its power to rule you; you're putting yourself in charge of it. Embrace it. Failing is far better than going stale in your career because you won't take a risk at doing something new.

- *Try something new.* After a mistake, be brave and try a completely different approach. You've heard of this quote attributed to Albert Einstein: "The definition of insanity is doing the same thing over and over again and expecting different results." Don't fall into that category. While it's OK to make mistakes, it's *not* OK to keep repeating the same mistakes. Do whatever it takes to prevent that from happening.

- *Reflect in the aftermath of failure.* Was your mistake a competency error? A political faux pas? The result of negligence? Do you need more training or practice? Do you need a better understanding of emotional intelligence and spheres of influence, for example? When you evaluate what happened, be honest with yourself. Think of the kinds of mistakes you tend to make and home in on the causes and solutions. Career advancement can be made on the heels of a mistake or a rejection (we discuss this point later), as long as you commit to learning from each failure and never repeating it.

TAKING AND HANDLING CRITICISM

Generally speaking, the higher your leadership position is, the more visible you are inside and outside the organization. The greater your visibility, the more critics you have and the more heat you must be willing to take. Everyone is scrutinizing your every move and feels entitled to share their opinions about your performance, decisions, behavior, character, associations or relationships, successes, and failures. You get called out for the things you did and didn't do. You get both wanted and unwanted, constructive and mean-spirited feedback. You get blamed for every problem and scolded for every solution that doesn't pan out. The negative attention can be relentless. And all of it happens privately and publicly, online and offline.

If you're uncomfortable with this barrage of criticism and feedback, now is a good time to grow thick skin and broad shoulders. You're gonna need them not only when you reach the C-suite but also as you make your way there. While we can't give you thick skin and broad shoulders, we can offer you advice on how to receive, view, and handle criticism, especially after a failure.

Essentially, people receive three kinds of criticisms: (1) angry or edgy comments that sting, admonish, demand, scare, shame, or belittle; (2) constructive feedback that informs, teaches, corrects, recommends improvements, points out weaknesses, and encourages; and (3) a combination of the two. Expect all kinds of criticism. Your boss may criticize you, and so may your team members and even complete strangers. As we said in chapter 8, step up to these difficult conversations.

When receiving criticism, be open and self-reflective. There's a little truth in everything. Don't immediately label as useless the feedback from a source you think has absolutely nothing to do with you. You might find nuggets of wisdom, no matter how tiny, in what that critic says. Don't dismiss the lessons from or the perspective of people you don't like or who are especially critical of you. Embrace all critiques and feedback. They give you fresh insights into, for example, why the failure took place, what areas you need to fix or approaches you need to adopt to prevent the same mistake, and how you can help yourself and others bounce back.

Three things can help you take and handle criticisms in general:

1.   *Personal development.* This includes but is certainly not limited to reading life-affirming books, listening to uplifting lectures or podcasts, and surrounding yourself with positive people. The happier you are, the less likely you are to be bothered by criticism.

2.   *Self-awareness.* Being aware of your strengths and weaknesses gives you confidence. It's not arrogance, but self-esteem—the feeling of being OK with who you are despite your flaws. This confidence allows you to process criticisms without getting emotionally and psychologically wrecked by the comments.

3.   *Coaching.* Many high performers rely on coaches. Elite athletes have position coaches, strength and conditioning coaches, and sports psychologists. Professional musicians

and vocalists have teachers and instructors. Leaders in various industries hire executive coaches. Why approach coaches instead of your sphere of influence for this purpose? Professional coaches provide objective inputs and resources, unlike biased and loyal friends and colleagues. Coaches routinely give feedback and critique elements of performance, making their clients immune to and responsive to the critique process. We're not saying those clients don't feel the sting and anxiety of regular criticism, but they have an acute understanding that the feedback is not a personal attack but a tool to coax their best performance.

See exhibit 9.1 for strategies for handling unsolicited criticism.

Exhibit 9.1 How to Handle Unsolicited Criticism

It's one thing to ask for and receive feedback from your network contacts and other work associates. But it's another to get unsolicited criticism. Resist the temptation to defend yourself. With the following steps, you can transform the negative into something productive:

- *Listen.* You may be quick to interrupt or state your case. Stop. Pay attention. Absorb what the person with the beef has to say. Wait for that person to finish, just as you would want if the tables were turned.

- *Consider the source.* Does this person have a genuine grievance? Or is he or she just jealous? Does this person have a track record of being insubordinate? To answer this question, you may need to reach out to your mentors, network contacts, or an objective party you respect. Ask them about the alleged critic and criticism. Find out if the criticism is truly justified.

- *Don't take it personally.* This may well be the hardest tip to follow. It's natural to take criticisms personally; after all, it's your brand on the line. Resist that urge. Maintain as much objectivity as you can. Otherwise, you won't get anything good out of this experience, only bad.

(continued)

- *Stay calm.* Take a deep breath. One of the worst things you can do is be reactive and lash out. You need presence of mind to explore whether or not the criticism is founded.

- *Ask clarifying questions.* If a blanket criticism is made ("You never respond to my e-mails!"), you'll feel like it doesn't hold much water. Ask for specifics, for details about where you allegedly went wrong. You can objectively judge if the criticism has merit only if you have these details. And you most certainly can't remedy the situation if you don't have the specifics about what you did wrong in the first place.

- *Take ownership.* If you really have wronged someone or some people, you need to own up to it. Apologize, and do it properly. (See chapter 4 for a longer discussion of apologies.) Personal accountability and humility are two hallmarks of exceptional leaders.

- *Embrace the message.* As a leader, you are in the seemingly counterintuitive position of valuing criticism. Because of your position, it's only natural that people will have a beef with you from time to time. You need to look at this as almost an honor, that people are so invested in the team or the organization they are willing to put themselves on the line to express that brash opinion. You just may have something to learn from this critique. You never know, there could be beautiful rewards in the end when you address the criticism.

- *Take action.* Yes, you need to do more than just nod and speak to the criticism. You need to act on it. Value the feedback or experience as an opportunity to grow professionally as a leader. If you grow from this difficult experience, you are unlikely to find yourself in the same situation again. Good for you, your team, and your entire organization.

Ultimately, how you respond to unsolicited criticism is what makes you stand out from other emerging leaders. Seize the opportunity to turn the negative into a positive.

PERSEVERING THROUGH THE NOS

You may not know who Cordia Harrington is, but chances are you know her product. Harrington's business, The Bakery Companies, makes the bread used by McDonald's, Kentucky Fried Chicken, and Chili's (among other major enterprises). This was not always the case, though. Harrington approached McDonald's 33 times before the restaurant chain said yes to her product. Thirty-three times!

How many nos do you need to hear before you stop asking the question? Before you throw in the proverbial towel? We'd bet that your threshold for rejection is lower than you think. That's because we live in an instant-gratification society, where if we don't get immediate results or an immediate yes, we get discouraged. If we get discouraged, we tend to give up.

But anything worth having is worth doing and is worth the wait, so keep going even when you hear that no, even if you're rejected many times. Persevere, as Harrington did; try other routes, as Laurie did (her story follows); and be gracious in the process, as Natalie was (see her story in this section as well).

Laurie's first healthcare job after college was as an administrative assistant in a large health system. She had no desire to stay in the role long term, so she started applying for roles both inside and outside the organization. In the two years she held the job, she was passed over for two internal promotions and two external interviews, both for entry-level management roles. If you're counting, that's four rejections! At this point she began to grow very discouraged. And impatient.

She could have thrown in the towel, but she stuck it out. In the end, her persistence resulted in a defining point in her career. Through a mentoring relationship she had developed, a seasoned executive offered her a role as vice president of clinics for a community hospital. She was 22 at the time. Landing the position more than tripled her salary. But more important, it gave her a priceless opportunity to advance her healthcare career and her leadership development.

The two years she endured getting rejected but refusing to back down felt like an eternity. But in reality, that period was barely more than a blip on the radar of her career.

When Natalie applied for her first CEO role, she initially was rejected. She wasn't considered for the final round of interviews because she lacked the five years of experience required for the job. When the hiring committee narrowed the field to four candidates, she was not selected as one of the four. Although disappointed, she took the decision in stride and wrote a follow-up thank-you note to the board and the hiring committee. The note impressed them, among other things.

Fast-forward two weeks. One of the candidates dropped out of contention and took another job, so the committee reached out to Natalie to give her an opportunity to interview. And she gave the interview of her young life. How did it turn out? Really well.

At 29 years old, Natalie became the CEO of a rural hospital. But had she adopted a defeatist, sour grapes attitude about the initial rejection, she might not have gotten a call back and might have missed out on her second chance.

Maximizing the Time in Between the No and the Yes

The first few years of your career seem to have a comparatively small impact on your overall career path, but this period is crucial to your development. It is the time to become stronger personally and professionally. It is the time to get tough. Ask yourself what you can do during this time to best position yourself when an opportunity comes along. Here are a few of our suggestions:

- *Be patient.* It's hard, *really* hard. Have confidence that your education, skills, and experiences have prepared you for the next level, but keep pursuing continual growth. Know that the right things will happen in your career when they're supposed to.
- *Look inward.* What are you doing with this experience? How do you apply the feedback and criticism you've received to better equip yourself for the next job? Instead of looking at others who seem to have it so easy, or even those who may

have landed the position you wanted, look inside you. See what you're doing to improve your chances of getting a yes. Often, a yes is simply beyond your control, but not always.

- *Work on your mental tenacity.* At some point during the 33 nos, Harrington probably wondered if something was wrong with her. We know how disheartening that must have been, and we experienced just a fraction of the rejection she was up against. But she held strong and has become an inspiration for (even the envy of) many entrepreneurs and fledgling executives. That's mental tenacity!

Mental tenacity is a rarely discussed trait of successful people, including leaders. It's not the same as mental discipline, which is being in control of how you think about and respond to situations (see chapter 5). It's the dogged, stubborn determination in the face of critics, naysayers, personal shortcomings, and other seemingly insurmountable obstacles. Tenacity is not about being emotionally bulletproof, as if your feelings don't get hurt when you fail or get rejected. It's about going for it anyway.

When you're mentally tenacious, you get better if you get a no. You don't surrender, you don't throw in the towel. One day, you can stash that towel away; you won't be needing it.

TRYING NEW THINGS

Somewhere around one year of age, most children try to walk. And after taking the first or second wobbly step (perhaps even before then), every one of those children falls. Some of them pick themselves back up like nothing happened, while others stay down and cry until they're ready to try again. They all go through this cycle of falling and getting up (and crying) many, many times. Then one day, success! They're walking—without wobbliness, without tears, without assistance from their parents. And then they move on to trying other things like running, going up and down stairs, climbing trees and tall objects, and riding a bike.

Children follow their natural curiosity. They find something of interest, and they explore it without fear of failure or pressure of success. How did we, as adults, lose so much of our childhood explorer mentality? Why are we so unwilling to risk trying new things, make mistakes or get rejected in the process, and recover only to try again?

If you've never failed, it doesn't mean you're better than everyone else. It means you're either incredibly lucky or not going beyond your comfort zone. If you want that dream job, go big! Get creative with your approach. Do something you've never done before. Explore all your options and try as many of them as possible. Don't be intimidated by failure, criticism, and rejection. Be brave and tenacious, just like a child learning to walk.

FORGETTING

Usually, forgetting (e.g., where we put our keys, the name of an old acquaintance) is considered a bad thing, a sign of advancing age or mental fogginess. But sometimes forgetting or selective memory can be an asset. Here's why.

After failure or rejection, bouncing back to performing at your highest level is much easier if you can forget (read: stop thinking about) what knocked you down in the first place. Remembering the details is critical during a debriefing and during self-reflection after the fact—so that you can trace where things went wrong and so that you don't do the same thing again. But beyond that, replaying the details in your mind every day acts as a distraction and a detriment to your efforts to move forward.

Think about it this way: If a quarterback remembers the game-losing interception he threw during a big game *each time* he passes the football, do you think he'll ever lead his team to the Super Bowl? If a nurse replays in her head that fateful day she administered the wrong dosage to a patient *each time* she hands out medications, do you think she'll ever gain back her confidence so as not to repeat the medical error?

Professionals move on. They have to so they can get back to doing what they love to do. If they don't, if they wallow in their failures or guilt or whatever psychological trauma they sustained, they will constantly second-guess themselves and weaken their performance. And poof, there goes their career.

As we said in the beginning of this chapter, you shouldn't define your career by your failures. You should define it by the way you overcame the adversity, by the way you bounced back and learned and thrived afterward.

Failure?! What failure?

Rookie Mistakes

Staying Psychologically Stuck

Failures can be devastating, as illustrated in this first-person account of Laurie's experience.

Shortly before the birth of my second child, I unexpectedly lost my company's only other employee under tragic circumstances. It was a tumultuous time, to say the least. I scrambled to perform and deliver for my clients, but ultimately I experienced some painful failures. And I let my clients down.

The workload spread between two employees now rested squarely on my eight-months'-pregnant shoulders. I was managing the construction project of a medical office building for a physician group client, and the completion date was a mere five weeks away. Another client was in the final stages

→

of recruiting a new physician and was revising its physician employment contract model.

During this time, I dropped a few balls, missed deadlines, and struggled to keep afloat. Seventy-two hours after the birth of my son, I was back in the office to meet a client's payroll audit deadline. I performed a construction punch list with a sleeping newborn in tow. Many of my clients were incredibly understanding and accommodating, but a few were less tolerant. Not delivering on a promise is unacceptable to me, because I'm a driven, Type A person. My credibility and my company's reputation are my livelihood.

Four months later, I added two new colleagues to the team, and my business started to experience tremendous growth. In fact, we were in the very fortunate position of being able to double the staff size again to meet demand. But for me, the residual impact of my recent failures remained. Instead of finding the positive in these experiences and then moving past the negative, I allowed the failures to linger and mushroom. They psychologically devastated me.

I felt like a failure. My self-worth took a significant hit. Just as my business was starting to gain some traction, I was losing ground. Simply put, I wasn't myself, and more important, I wasn't the leader the company needed at the time.

During these years, I was wrestling with the desire to pursue new business opportunities and devote myself more exclusively to speaking and training. I kept thinking that if we just grew a bit more I would be freed up to do my own thing.

One word: delusional.

Despite our growth, I started to make decisions based on emotion. I was losing objectivity. I allowed one significant event

→

to grab hold of me and let it dictate everything, when circumstances demanded stellar, committed, confident leadership.

Ultimately, I ended up dismantling the atomic bomb. I divested two major client relationships to two of my employees, who went on to form their own practice management consultancy. My other three employees accepted healthcare leadership roles elsewhere in the community. By the end of the following year, the transitions were complete. Without focus and passion for the company in its current construct, I was not capable of guiding its continued growth.

Now, I *know* that failures don't define us. And failures certainly aren't final—if you don't let them become the be-all, end-all. That truth, my friends, is easier said than lived. Unfortunate circumstances resulting in mistakes are as inevitable as taxes. Sure they hurt, but you've got to keep going regardless. Don't allow them to bring you down—at least not for long—because out of these challenges come opportunities to rise above in a way that, perhaps, wouldn't have been possible had you not developed the fortitude from a major setback.

Remember These

- Failures are a matter of *when*, never a matter of *if*. All we can do is hope for the best, but plan for the worst.
- Don't define your career in this constantly changing, high-stress, high-stakes healthcare industry by the number of times you failed or made a mistake. How you overcome or rebound from adversity is what should

→

define your career, because that's tough work that not only requires but also shows your strength of character.

- Failure is good because it provides learning and growth opportunities. It also promotes taking risks by applying new approaches to old or existing processes.

- The higher your leadership position is, the more visible you are inside and outside the organization. The greater your visibility, the more critics you have and the more heat you must be willing to take.

- Don't dismiss the lessons from or the perspective of people you don't like or who are especially critical of you. Embrace all critiques and feedback.

- Anything worth having is worth doing and is worth the wait, so keep going even when you hear that no, even if you're rejected many times.

- If you've never failed, it doesn't mean you're better than everyone else. It means you're either incredibly lucky or not going beyond your comfort zone.

REFERENCE

Kalb, I. 2013. "Innovation Isn't Just About Brainstorming New Ideas." *Business Insider*. Published July 8. www.businessinsider.com/innovate-or-die-a-mantra-for-every-business-2013-7.

CHAPTER 10

Network, Network, Network!

Surround yourself with only people who are
going to lift you higher.

—*Oprah Winfrey, TV personality*

Reading Points

- Networking Done Right

- Networking for Introverts

- Network Up

- Networking According to Your Season of Life

SOME PROFESSIONALS MIGHT think that networking is a luxury
they can't afford. "I'm too busy as it is!" they might say, justifying
their decision to skip an industry event in which they could connect with hundreds of people. But networking is far from a luxury.
It's a basic necessity that professionals can't afford to do without.

Want to raise your visibility and profile in your organization
and beyond? You must network. Want to get the inside scoop on a
position, change disciplines or enter a different field, get job offers,
or make a lateral or vertical career move? You must network. Want

to be introduced or exposed to those whose career path you admire? You must network. Plus, continual networking (read: developing rapport and serving your contacts) is beneficial even when you already have a job or don't have a specific need. Someday, you will need to tap into this network, and the relationships you've been building will already be there to lend you a hand.

Don't think that networking is only beneficial for early careerists and job seekers. It's also a go-to activity for mid-level professionals and senior executives who are continual learners, relationship builders, people persons, collaborators, communicators, innovators, strategists, and doers. They fully engage with their network for all kinds of reasons—from exchanging and testing ideas to discovering new approaches to problem solving to forming partnerships, to name just a few. (See exhibit 10.1 for two examples of how a simple networking relationship can evolve into a job offer and a partnership.)

Exhibit 10.1 Networking = More Working

From Colleague to Boss

For nine out of the ten years Laurie owned a consulting firm, she shared clients with John, a bank president. While she assisted her physician clients in launching their private practices, he assisted these same clients with their practices' financing and banking needs. He earned their business nearly every time, presenting strong responses to the requests for proposals and delivering valuable industry expertise and stellar customer service.

The two had mutual clients and worked on many shared projects over the years. During that time, Laurie's consultancy focus transitioned from healthcare management to leadership development and strengths-based leadership facilitation. John engaged her to work with his executive team and to facilitate a strengths retreat. Eventually, he offered to acquire a portion of her business and to create within his organization a unique position custom-made for Laurie. She would lead the bank's brand strategy, organizational culture, and healthcare banking division. The opportunity, though nontraditional, was a brilliant fit, bolstered by their mutual respect for each other's expertise, their rapport, and their years of supporting each other's business. Laurie jumped at the offer.

(continued)

She didn't apply for the job; in fact, she wasn't even looking for jobs at all. Her consistent networking approach, however, brought her this opportunity and steered her toward a career path she never could have defined on her own.

When Natalie Met Laurie

In the spring of 2008, Laurie and Natalie were both attendees at the American College of Healthcare Executives (ACHE) Leaders Conference in Phoenix. On day one of the conference, the presenter asked all 35 attendees to stand up one by one to introduce themselves. When Natalie got up and told the room she was the CEO of a hospital, Laurie thought, "Wow, she looks about my age. I need to introduce myself and get to know her." That afternoon during the coffee break, Laurie did just that. They made plans to connect over dinner the following evening. They had a great conversation at dinner, and they both enjoyed and learned a lot from each other. On day three of the conference, they parted ways, having exchanged business cards.

One week later, Laurie called Natalie's office.

"Hey, this is Laurie Baedke. We just met in Phoenix, but would you have any interest in collaborating with me on an ACHE Congress session for early careerists around the concepts of professional development, networking, and career path design?"

"Is this that blonde woman I had dinner with last week?" Natalie thought to herself. Aloud she said, "I'm interested, but when is it due? Tell me more!"

Inspiration was sparked and a plan was drafted. Three weeks later, they submitted a session proposal for Congress 2009. It was accepted. Now, nine years later, the session is alive and well. It has even become this book.

Big business (as well as small business) is also in the networking game. Think Walmart, with its network of suppliers and distributors; Amazon, with its network of warehouses; and Apple, with its network of iTunes customers. These corporations all leverage their networks. As a result, they achieve something far more powerful than what each entity could do on its own.

The same applies to you. With your network, you can accomplish things more quickly, more efficiently, and more effectively, and you can go farther than you can alone. More heads are definitely better than one.

Now here's the most important thing to remember about networking: Don't go into networking counting and anticipating all the advantages or benefits you will gain from each connection. Instead, focus on how you can be of service to those people or how you can help them achieve their goals. Your rewards (including the intangible goodwill and shared learning) will come naturally, organically, later or when you least expect them. Interestingly, those who don't think of their own personal gain always seem to end up getting the most from networking. Isn't that ironic?

In this chapter, we cover various aspects of networking, including the patience required to develop and nurture relationships, the kind of people you should add to your network, and strategies for introverts and for networking up.

NETWORKING DONE RIGHT

Networking is not about collecting business cards at cocktail receptions or taking new contacts out for lunch or coffee and then forgetting all about them until you have to ask a favor or a question and then disappearing from their life again until you need something—and then rinse, repeat. That's the surest way to make people feel used and thus to disassociate from you altogether. They might do as you requested the first time (perhaps to be nice), but you won't hear from them again the next time you come calling.

So what should you do to get this right? Following are some of our suggestions. These practices might seem like common sense, but they rarely are practiced. Do them without fail throughout your career, and you will create a network so rich and robust that it can lead to and sustain your career success.

Develop and Maintain Lasting Relationships

Treat networking as a lifestyle, something you do regularly as a habit, not as a one-time effort. Send notes and cards to thank people for spending time with you recently. Make phone calls to check in. E-mail a link to an article that you know they are interested in (professionally or personally). Meet them when you're in their town (or vice versa) or when you're both at a social or professional event. Like, comment on, or share their social media posts. Support their initiatives. Extend an offer to help before they ask or even if they don't ask. Get to know them personally (respecting their boundaries, of course), and remember some details about them that you can bring up the next time you see each other. Introduce them to others you think they may be interested in getting to know.

These little acts add up and help you build a lasting relationship with every member of your network. They show you care about them and your connection. They show your strength of character. They show you are there to serve their needs and interests, not the other way around.

Because of the rapport you're establishing, in the future you may feel less awkward or uncomfortable about, for example, approaching a CEO contact for a job recommendation or asking a colleague for information that is not readily accessible (e.g., if a coveted position will soon open because of unforeseen staffing changes).

Be Patient

Networking is a lot of things, but fast it is not. No instant gratification here. But that's to be expected. After all, no one can build a lasting relationship in a few hours, weeks, or even months. If you want to do networking right, you must invest time into it (read:

years, even decades), and you have to practice patience. This means you have to continually meet people, earn their trust and respect, get to know them, pay attention to their needs, and serve them or make them look good—all without expecting anything in return. Again, network when you don't need to network (just like you should look for a job when you don't need a job). Your network will be there for you to draw from when you do need it for whatever reason—big or small—and through seasons of your life when it is not your top priority.

If you don't put in the time and patience, you may be creating superficial, short-term connections in which everyone involved is just in it to use everyone else and then burn all bridges. This should go without saying, but burning bridges is never, ever a good move. Healthcare is a small world. You never know where you could end up later in your career. The people you offend, take advantage of, mistreat, or abandon today might be the same people you could be working for or who could be offering you a golden opportunity tomorrow.

Diversify Your Network

Connect with stellar people inside and outside your industry and area of expertise. For example, you could network with clinicians, academics and educators, business leaders, consumer advocates, healthcare quality researchers, health policymakers, and patient groups. Plus, you could network with the following:

- Your mentors
- Rising stars and centers of influence in your organization
- Thought leaders in your industry and other related industries (e.g., pharmaceutical, long-term care)
- Former colleagues

- Former professors and classmates as well as alumni from your undergraduate and graduate programs
- Peers and emerging leaders in your community or industry
- Staff of your professional associations
- Representatives from your civic and charitable organizations (e.g., nonprofits, faith-based groups, parent–teacher associations, chambers of commerce, and Rotary clubs)

The point is to surround yourself with a good mix of people—in terms of gender, age or generation, geography, industry, education and training, ethnicity or cultural background, and so on. Fostering a diverse network exposes you to various styles, walks of life, perspectives, areas of expertise, and bodies of knowledge that help cultivate your well-roundedness and open-mindedness. This way, you are not isolated from other disciplines and your influence extends beyond your field.

Be Selective

Speaking of influence, remember the *average five* theory we discussed in chapter 7? It is the idea that the five people you spend the most time with shape and influence you, and you in turn shape and influence five more people, and on the cycle goes. Because of this influence, you and those closest to you share the same beliefs, mentality, and even hobbies or interests. They also reflect, in general, your health, financial, and career status.

The professionals in your network exert the same kind of influence on you, so be cautious when selecting your associates. Pick people who are like-minded and can reinforce or support your growth (and vice versa). Stay away from those who are negative and whose career choices or reputation could hurt yours. Serving them could prove challenging.

Be Consistent

Consistency is key in good leadership and in good networking. Think about your favorite supervisor or manager. Chances are she or he gives you feedback—both positive and negative—on a regular basis and not just when something goes wrong or during your annual evaluation. The manager is consistent and methodical with giving you input and asking you to make adjustments when needed. This way, you always know not only how you're performing your duties but also where you stand with the manager and what is expected of you. Best of all, you get no surprises.

Networking should be treated with the same consistent strategy. Not only should you keep engaging with the people in your network (and doing so selflessly), but you should also keep seizing new opportunities to network (see exhibit 10.2). Otherwise, one day you might be shocked to find that the network you've built over many years has diminished in both strength and number.

Last but not least: Make sure your offline (or "real-life" self) and online personas are consistent with each other. Be authentic or be your true self regardless of whether you're interacting with your network on social media or face-to-face. Displaying two different personalities or pretending you're more or other than who you are will confuse your audience and make them think you are playing games at best and are untrustworthy at worst.

Exhibit 10.2 Seven Strategies for Growing Your Network

Valuable resources are all around you, and with just a little bit of legwork you can easily tap into them. Take the initiative to seek out new networking relationships whenever you can. Here are just a few ways:

1. *Work your alumni network.* Whether you are still a student, just graduated, or finished your degree decades ago, you can check out your college's/university's rich directory of alumni. Most schools keep good tabs on their high-performing former students and can connect

(continued)

you with them. From this directory, you can find a potential mentor or a networking partner in your geographic area or area of interest.

2. *Launch an internal search.* Identify those in your organization who have political capital and reach out to them. These individuals may be up-and-coming leaders or colleagues who may be a step or two ahead of you career-wise. Whatever the case may be, asking them individually to join you for a 30-minute coffee break or a 1-hour lunch conversation can go a long way.

3. *Get involved in your community.* Choose a local cause that is near and dear to your heart—anything from a grassroots movement to a young professionals civic group to a nonprofit organization. Call and ask how you can volunteer. Doing so enables you to stay informed about the issues in your community, serve other people, hone skills that you may not use on a daily basis, develop personally, and meet people and build relationships. Volunteering will give more to you than you give to it. That's a fact.

   Healthcare leadership volunteering is also possible. For example, Laurie's mentor encouraged her to sit on the board of her local ACHE chapter in Nebraska. She was only two years into her career, so she thought, "What could I possibly have to offer?" Her volunteer service meant doing event planning, managing contacts, hosting speakers, and other grunt work. Not glamorous, but personally and professionally very rewarding. Volunteering afforded her a fantastic opportunity to connect with many influential healthcare leaders in the area.

4. *Become a card-carrying member of professional associations.* Industry organizations give you opportunities to meet local and national healthcare leaders, to share and learn best practices in various areas of healthcare management, and to lead or participate in discussions about industry issues, among other benefits. Plus, you get to connect with like-minded professionals who are on a similar career path or in the same season of life as you. Reach out to the local chapter of these associations. Their representatives can help you get started. (See exhibit 10.3 for more discussion on association membership.)

5. *Take advantage of social media and other online resources.* If you're not yet *professionally* active online, start. Now. This goes beyond having a passive account on LinkedIn, Twitter, Facebook, and other social media platforms. It involves active engagement, including following trusted thought leaders, movers and shakers, pioneers and innovators, and organizational leaders; sharing industry-related news, research and case studies, journal articles, and other informative tidbits with your connections; writing healthcare-related posts (long or short) that stimulate dialogue between you and

(continued)

readers; and hosting or participating in virtual discussions about topics that affect the industry. Doing so can quickly build your professional online presence, and pretty soon it will lead to new contacts that you can nurture into networking relationships.

6. *Introduce yourself.* At events, step out of your comfort zone. Don't default to sitting with your friends or existing contacts for the whole day. That doesn't do you or them any favor. Catch up with them before or after (or whatever works for you), but excuse yourself during the event so that you (and they) can meet and mingle with other attendees, session presenters, lead speakers, exhibitors (who are not just vendors but representatives of organizations), and so on. Arrive early or stay late to maximize your time, if you must. Introducing yourself to strangers may be uncomfortable and nerve-wracking, but remember that just about everyone there is in the same situation as you and is feeling the same thing. And we assure you that the vast majority of people at these events are pleasant and receptive to networking with you.

   Let's go back to introducing yourself to the speaker. Before the speaker's presentation, approach him or her; you could *briefly* mention who you are and why you're looking forward to the talk, and you could ask whether you might contact him or her in the future should you have any follow-up questions or if you could be of service. By doing this, you're making your presence known to a well-respected and influential person (otherwise he or she wouldn't be presenting in the first place!), and you're opening lines of communication between the two of you (which could lead to a mentorship or networking relationship). The speaker may reference you as an example during the presentation, which would be a bonus because it will increase your visibility and help you make more connections during the event.

7. *Help others build their network.* If you're consistent enough to have developed a robust network, take the initiative to introduce pairs of people you know to each other, if you think they would be good partners and would gain mutual benefits. Call it network matchmaking. For example, do you know a professor looking desperately for a research assistant? Do you also know a student or a new careerist aspiring to be in academia? Voilà, you have a match! Introduce them to each other. These pairings may not always work, but the point is you're exercising the value of your network and making that network valuable for others as well. And the more you help others, the better your reputation gets, the more connections come your way, the more you can help, and so on. Good begets good; don't forget that.

Exhibit 10.3 Association Membership

A decade ago, the William E. Smith Institute for Association Research published the findings of a study on association membership. The report revealed that association members earn more, like their jobs more, and are even happier than people who do not belong to any association (Brooks 2008). Because the research was done for the association community, these results are likely biased, so take them with a grain of salt. That being said, our personal experience and recommendation align with this research.

But do note: Simply being a member and paying your annual dues will not lead to the well-connected career you want, just as merely having a gym membership will not lead to the strong body you want. You must take advantage of the resources and privileges available to you. You must actively engage to get as much value out of that association as you can.

Following is a short list (certainly not all-inclusive) of healthcare associations we suggest you look into:

- American College of Healthcare Executives (ACHE)
- American Health Care Association (AHCA)
- American Hospital Association (AHA)
- Asian Healthcare Leaders Forum (AHLF)
- Healthcare Financial Management Association (HFMA)
- Healthcare Information and Management Systems Society (HIMSS)
- Medical Group Management Association (MGMA)
- National Association of Health Services Executives (NAHSE)
- National Association of Latino Healthcare Executives (NALHE)
- Specialization associations (e.g., American Association of Orthopaedic Executives, American Academy of Ophthalmic Executives, Association for Directors of Radiation Oncology Programs)

Plus, you can check out young professionals (YP) groups in your community as well as local or industry leadership programs (e.g., Leadership Omaha).

Present Yourself as a Memorable and Genuine Professional

Your personal and professional selves (the things you can change and manage) combined with your reputation (the things others say about you that you cannot control) make up your personal brand (see chapter 6). The *you* brand is what others see when you network. You must present it in a memorable and genuine fashion. Here are some tips on how you can set yourself apart among your contacts:

- *Dress and conduct yourself as if you are already holding the position you desire.* Always be aware of the nature and location of the networking event and dress appropriately. If the setting is casual, be on the sharper edge of business casual. You won't find too many healthcare CEOs, for example, in jeans and a fleece or in ill-fitted khakis and a golf shirt. If you're unsure, find out the dress code.

  Don't be memorable for the wrong reasons. Be remembered as the one person who wore a tailored suit, not as the one who drank too much at the reception and spoke too loudly and told inappropriate jokes. Regardless of how casual the networking event is, you don't have permission to behave unprofessionally or to forget all the rules of social decorum. You are there to spark new professional relationships and invest in existing ones. You are not there to draw negative attention to yourself or be the life of the party; that behavior may only garner you an embarrassing mention in someone's blog, tweet, Facebook post, or LinkedIn update—or worse, a red flag in the memory of a key center of influence.

  Be polite, willing to participate in activities, friendly, and approachable. You don't have to be perky, but you should be positive (not sarcastic, cynical, or a contrarian).

You don't have to be the most intelligent person in the room or know everything, but you should be able to hold a conversation about a host of topics (including healthcare trends) with a diverse group. And you don't have to be the best talker, but you should be an active listener; this entails not just nodding your head but also asking follow-up questions and occasionally relating to what is being said.

- *Be a genuine connector.* Introducing your associates to those you believe they ought to know and then getting out of their way is one of the surest ways to show that you're genuine about serving others, that you're not in the relationship just to benefit you, and that you're looking out for their interests. If you're only pretending to care, your contacts will see right through it. For example, if you strongly urge a current colleague to interview with a hiring manager you know from another organization in the guise of helping the coworker practice her interviewing skills, but in reality your plot is to push her out because you secretly want her position, then your behavior and intentions are purely selfish. When (not *if*) your colleague finds out what you're doing, she could hurt your reputation. And thanks to the Internet, word travels fast. It takes a long time to rebuild your brand after this kind of offense.

- *Stay informed, and be thoughtful.* On top of sending handwritten notes for various purposes (e.g., saying thanks, congratulations, or just a hello), keep yourself updated on what your associates are doing. Set up Google alerts for the leading organizations and individuals in your network. Check your connections' LinkedIn updates. Read association newsletters and trade magazines. Did anyone publish an article, switch jobs or get promoted, win an award or a notable honor, earn a certification, pass an exam, launch a business or a product, or participate in a successful initiative? Use this knowledge to reach out and make a warm contact. How would you feel if someone you once connected with, but hadn't touched based with in a while, sent you a surprise e-mail congratulating you on a recent promotion? It would be a memorable moment, that's for sure. And all it took was a minute of that person's time.

Staying informed can also help you leave a great impression—and that's a plus for a new careerist. For example, when your CEO asks if anyone is aware of proposed hospital legislation in a neighboring state and its potential implication for your organization, you're going to want to know exactly what the CEO's talking about and to be able to share your opinion.

Finally, remember the things that are important to your contacts, and bring them up in your conversation. How are your twin three-year-old granddaughters? Are you still volunteering at the women's shelter? Have you finished building that boat with your son? Teddy Roosevelt's quote, "People don't care how much you know, until they know how much you care," rings true here.

NETWORKING FOR INTROVERTS

The best networkers are extroverts, right? We beg to differ.

We believe that being self-aware and being consistent at networking trump differences in personality. You don't have to be gregarious or a social butterfly, flitting from one group to the next, to attract contacts. You can be shy or reserved and still build lasting networking relationships. The key is to know how you operate. Do you prefer e-mails and notes to phone calls and face-to-face? Are you more comfortable with one-on-one than with group activity? Does the idea of entering a circle of strangers to introduce yourself terrify you? Once you understand these and other things about yourself, you can develop your own networking approach. Although the recommendations we present in this chapter offer something for both introverts and extroverts, we urge you to create an approach that works best for you. (Note that the advice we give here may apply to everybody, not just introverts.)

Whatever you do, don't skip networking events just because you don't think you could handle them. Go! Show up! Practice introducing yourself in the mirror, over and over and over until you become masterful (or at least proficient) at it. Work on your elevator speech—that is, what you'd like to say about yourself—and questions you'd like to ask when you meet someone new. Don't approach crowds, if you're uncomfortable; strike up a conversation with an individual and then move on to another. Don't forget to exchange business cards, as you'll want to follow up later to thank the person for the chat or to fill in the blanks that you might have forgotten in your nervous state. And if you write well, wow your new contacts with a sincere note; you could make a good impression that way, if you thought you didn't during your initial meeting.

Social media can also help. Before the event, reach out to a few of your contacts via LinkedIn, Twitter, or Facebook. Prime the pump, so to speak. Let them know you're looking forward to finally meeting face-to-face. This will make the meeting much more comfortable, efficient, and effective.

Networking is not a talent or a character trait. It's a skill you can learn that doesn't require you to become someone you're not. All it needs is your consistent input.

NETWORK UP

Heard of the term *marry up*? Now let's introduce you to the concept of *network up*. By this we mean keep company with the big boys and girls, the wise, the real deals. Soon enough, you'll become the company you keep.

We're not talking about hanging out with chief executives or senior-level managers (although you should approach them as well). We're talking about surrounding yourself with high performers and high achievers (no matter their organizational titles or rank). These are people who have a strong work ethic, who are ambitious and driven, who are disciplined and tenacious, who make things happen, who try even at the risk of failure and embarrassment, and who bring their A game all the time—and insist you do, too. A network filled with these types of people may be intimidating initially because they can be demanding and make your nerves dance a little bit, but they will inspire you to be better at everything you do.

Face it: Being the best of the bottom of the barrel is not a compliment. It might make others view you as a slacker by association. And that's a toxic perception, especially when you're just starting out and trying to prove yourself. So, as we said earlier, select your associates carefully.

It's natural for you to think you're not good enough, at this early stage, to associate with the movers and shakers, but snap out of it! Stretch yourself, and don't let any naysayers stop you. You'll steadily gain confidence once you realize that these people are receptive to you. That's the first step. The second step is to seek out these high achievers and connect with them. Look around your department, organization, community, and industry to identify those whose character, style, skills, and knowledge impress you. The rest of the steps are all up to you.

Five Benefits of Networking Up

1. *Learning opportunity.* When you fill your sphere of influence with wise professionals, you will inevitably learn something—from their successes, mistakes or failures, experiences, and daily habits. It's up to you to observe, listen for, and absorb the lessons. The reverse is true, too.

If you find that your network comprises people who are comfortable with the status quo and the mediocre and who don't care whether you succeed or fail, then you'll learn those negative habits.

2. *Better accountability.* When you network up, you are also signing yourself up to be accountable for whatever goals you set for yourself. These people are driven to achieve, so they expect the same from you. Suddenly, you've got a network of people holding you responsible for your own good. They will check on your progress, motivate and encourage you, shoot down every one of your excuses, give you advice and tools (even tough love), help you put things in perspective when you're faced with big decisions and barriers or if you fall short, and then challenge you to try again and again. With this kind of support, you'll have no excuse to give up or to not take your own growth seriously.

3. *Source of inspiration.* Even though the associates you admire and want to emulate are not perfect, they are inspirational to you anyway. If you spend enough time with them, you'll find yourself doing what they do, doing what they ask or imply, and doing the right thing. That's what happens in general when you connect with people you see as role models and as guides or teachers. Their actions, experiences, accomplishments, and wisdom compel you to follow their lead and to strive to be as good.

4. *Reason to stretch yourself.* Networking up may feel like you're in a secret competition with your connections. This motivates you to step up your game to catch up with, keep up with, or outpace their moves. This healthy challenge is a good thing, and even fun! The more you stretch yourself, the better you get (even if you fail). The better you get, the more opportunities (networking or otherwise) come your way. And the more opportunities come your way, the closer you get to your goals.

5. *Exercise in humility.* Amid all these high performers, inspiration, and competitors, it's impossible not to feel humbled. After all, you're surrounded by people who have stellar brands and whose reputation precedes them. Humility works two ways here. First, you're humbled by the caliber of the people around you. Second, you're humbled by the fact that you have a lot more growing up and learning to do, by your network's generosity in mentoring or teaching you—regardless of whether they do it deliberately or unintentionally—and by the lack of self-awareness and abundance of ego you've displayed in the past when you thought you had already arrived.

Board of Career Advisors

From your network of high performers, you can select the members of what we call a *board of career advisors* (aka sphere of influence, which is discussed in earlier chapters). These are people you trust to keep your confidences, to serve as a sounding board for your ideas and concerns, to give you honest feedback, and to advise you on various professional matters. They don't necessarily have to be friends, but they could include acquaintances, friends, and even family members. Most important, they must exercise discretion (as you will). This is a must, not an option.

Embrace your board of career advisors, and serve its members with TLC. But remember to be careful about what and how much you divulge. There is no place for TMI (too much information) in leadership, although it may be tempting to let your guard down once you get closer to certain members of your board. You have to strike a delicate balance. On the one hand, you want to be authentic and share everything (including organizational information few people have access to), but on the other hand, you have a responsibility to keep things professional and at arm's length. If you assemble a board of trustworthy, mature people, though, you can rest assured they will understand where you're coming from. (This board concept is discussed more in chapter 11.)

NETWORKING ACCORDING TO YOUR SEASON OF LIFE

Your networking approach and needs will differ depending on the season of your life. At the beginning of your career, perhaps without the obligations of a spouse or young children, investing heavily in your networking efforts may come easily. But as your seasons change (e.g., when you get married, raise a family, take on more responsibilities at work), your ability to attend evening networking events, weekend community volunteer activities, or leadership or association engagements may become limited. These obligations and commitments could force you to be more strategic in how you invest in networking.

That's totally OK. Normal and expected, even. Embrace the seasons of your life and network accordingly. Just don't stop networking entirely. No matter how much or how little time you dedicate to networking, be intentional about what you choose to participate in.

Evaluate your goals and objectives every once in a while to see if your time is being invested in a manner that nets a productive outcome. Consider what you commit to and what you don't. Every *yes* you say means a *no* to something else. Make it clear to those you say *no* to that it simply means "not now" and not forever.

The lesson is to network consistently and as much as you can early in your career, before family and other obligations become your highest priorities. Again, this is a tiny act with a compounding effect. That is, every "deposit" you make into your networking bank adds up. First, it establishes a positive habit. And later, when you can't network as much, you can "withdraw" from this bank, allowing you to still take advantage of your earlier efforts.

Remember These

- With your network, you can accomplish things more quickly, more efficiently, and more effectively and you can go farther than you can alone.
- Don't go into networking counting and anticipating all the advantages or benefits you will gain from each connection. Instead, focus on how you can be of service to those people or how you can help them achieve their goals.
- Treat networking as a lifestyle, something you do regularly as a habit, not as a one-time effort.
- If you want to do networking right, you must invest time into it (read: years, even decades).
- Fostering a diverse network exposes you to various styles, walks of life, perspectives, areas of expertise, and bodies of knowledge that help cultivate your well-roundedness and open-mindedness.
- The professionals in your network exert the same kind of influence on you, so be cautious when selecting your associates. Pick people who are like-minded and can reinforce or support your growth (and vice versa).
- Not only should you keep engaging with the people in your network (and doing so selflessly), but you should also keep seizing new opportunities to network.
- Being self-aware and being consistent at networking trump differences in personality. You don't have to be gregarious or a social butterfly to attract contacts. You can be shy or reserved and still build lasting networking relationships.

$\rightarrow$

- Network up: Surround yourself with high performers and high achievers. Soon enough, you'll become the company you keep.

- Your networking approach and needs will differ depending on the season of your life. No matter how much or how little time you dedicate to networking, be intentional about what you choose to participate in.

REFERENCE

Brooks, A. C. 2008. *Where Winners Meet: Why Happier, More Successful People Gravitate Toward Associations*. Published January. www.melosinstitute.org/Resources/Documents/Smith%20Buck%20Where%20Winners%20Meet.pdf.

Note to My 25-Year-Old Self

The first thing I would tell my 25-year-old self is to maintain a proper perspective, enjoy every moment, and view all challenges as opportunities. The most valuable lessons to be learned will come from opportunities you create and experiences you have. You will face both positive and challenging situations and outcomes. But all these experiences—in combination with a focus on your mission, objectives, and a desire to be true to yourself—will be key in shaping and developing values and a leadership character that will guide your path. Examples of opportunities to create and gain positive experiences include working with mentors; gaining insight into management structure, operations, strategic thinking, and decision making; working collaboratively with professionals who embrace learning; and having the independent responsibility that leads to your further growth. Additionally, some of your experiences will include managing through situations you have no control over, dealing with management styles you do not agree with, accepting decisions that are opposite to your position, and encountering conflict.

As you develop from a young professional into a manager and then a seasoned leader, realize the value of open-mindedness, understand that no one management style or decision is the definitive method or answer, approach life and work with your youthful but mature energy and enthusiasm, listen and see, and be inquisitive and ask questions.

What you will come to learn is the value of all experiences, including those that were not so positive but, when put in proper perspective, helped shape and define your character and leadership approach, which will be your framework to success and will keep you true to yourself.

Signed,
Christine M. Candio, RN, FACHE
Chairman (2014–2015), American College of Healthcare Executives
President and CEO, St. Luke's Hospital

CHAPTER 11

Engage a Mentor, Be a Mentor

If I hadn't had mentors, I wouldn't be here today. I'm a
product of great mentoring, great coaching. . . . Coaches or
mentors are very important. They could be anyone—your
husband, other family members, or your boss.

—Indra Nooyi, CEO, PepsiCo

Reading Points

- Identifying a Mentor

- Putting Together a Board of Career Advisors

- Getting Started

- Giving Back to the Field

WHAT COMES TO mind when you think of a mentor? Chances
are you envision someone a couple of decades older than you,
someone with a senior leadership title or in a position of power, or
someone well known in the community. But, in reality, a mentor
is not as out of reach as you may imagine. She or he can come from
all walks of life and is likely already playing an important role in
your life or career; it could even be you—to someone else, that is.

Although no definitive guideline exists for who a mentor should be or what a mentoring relationship should entail, all mentors share a clear and known characteristic: They enrich your life by contributing to your personal growth and/or professional development. How do they do this? By serving as your teacher, role model, sounding board, cheerleader, support system, devil's advocate, helping hand, confidant, and so on.

Specifically, mentors can

- *help you realize your full potential.* This is really at the heart of mentoring. Mentors see the potential in you, and they do what they can to nudge (even push) you toward becoming the person or professional you could be. They point you to resources for developing your natural abilities and aptitudes.

- *set an example.* Experienced professionals carry a hefty toolkit full of tools (e.g., advice, methods, strategies, tactics, solutions) they have picked up throughout their career. As mentors, they willingly share these tools and stories of their mistakes. The goal is to make their experiences into examples so that you can avoid the same mistakes they committed and stay on the right path.

- *provide honest feedback.* As an early careerist, you need to surround yourself with individuals who don't soothe and coddle your ego all the time and thus are not afraid to "tell it like it is." An honest mentor understands that a candid critique will strengthen your character, skills, and performance better than nonstop praise (which may not always be genuine) and agreement can ever do.

- *extend opportunities.* Experienced mentors, by virtue of the professional clout they've amassed over the years, may be in a position to leverage their contacts and reputation for your benefit. This opens career doors for you to walk or run through.

- *help you understand yourself better.* Great mentors ask questions. Then, they listen for the answers and probe with follow-up questions. By doing so, they help you become more self-aware, which is a foundation for your success.
- *challenge your status quo.* Mentors push you out of your comfort zone by presenting perspectives you hadn't considered before, challenging you to stretch yourself, assuring you that it's OK to fail and make mistakes, and encouraging you to try something new.

In this chapter, we walk you through the basics of mentorship. We cover the hows of identifying a mentor and assembling a board of career advisors, the whys of serving your board and mentor, and the when of giving back to the field.

IDENTIFYING A MENTOR

Visualize the position you'd like to fill, the kind of person and leader you'd like to be, and the influence you'd like to have on others in the future. Observe people who today are in the exact place you want to be in tomorrow. Note what they do and why, how they interact with and serve others, what skills and experiences they have, what their reputation is among others, who their mentors are and who makes up their network or sphere of influence, how self-aware they are, what career path they took (or are taking) to reach their ultimate goals, whether they're continual learners and willing teachers (especially to up-and-comers), and so on. If you like what you see, then you can approach one or two of those people to be your mentor (you don't have to limit yourself to one).

Don't be afraid to ask a CEO or senior executive. They were in your shoes once, so they'll be able to relate to your early career experiences and mentoring needs. But don't limit your search for a mentor to the C-suite, either. Look around and explore other avenues, if your regular network does not connect you to a mentor. Here are our recommendations:

1. Turn to your alumni network for slightly older peers—those only two or three years ahead of you—who are still amid their early-career struggles or challenges and thus can offer you timely and relevant insights and guidance.

2. Scan your organization for the rising stars (e.g., young managers, project leads, mid-level employees)—those whose names you hear often and who have earned the trust, respect, and admiration of the internal and external people they've worked with. The excellent job they do and their reputation expose them to diverse experiences, opportunities, people, approaches, and challenges. You can learn a lot from them.

3. Join a professional or charitable board in your community, or volunteer for a local cause you support. There, you'll find a mix of individuals from whom you can glean out-of-industry perspectives and advice that are applicable to your life and work.

4. Serve your boss and profession. Both are enormous resources. Your boss is already serving as your daily teacher, and if you make her or him look good (by being the reliable go-to person), you will learn even more. Association membership and events are mentorship (not just networking) mines. The more you develop yourself professionally, the more visibility you gain in the field and the better your chances of attracting the mentors who suit you.

The Authenticity Factor

Authenticity is a big factor in an effective mentoring relationship. As a mentee, you can't expect to get helpful advice and guidance from your mentor if you aren't honest about yourself and your concerns, worries, goals, and dreams. Your mentor will find it hard to get through to you if you are pretending to be someone you're not. Be open about your faults and shortcomings, and accept responsibility for fixing or improving them. Allow yourself to be groomed, to be taught, to be criticized, and to be challenged. Embrace your role as the student, and absorb as much as you can.

Choose a mentor who is also willing to be genuine, honest, and open with you. Mutual sharing of triumphs is great, but mutual sharing of defeats is a must. After all, stories about failures, embarrassments, or disappointments resonate louder than stories about wins and accomplishments. The latter type may be more inspiring, but the former type (though it might not be obvious) is more real, relatable, humbling, and educational. It reminds us no one's career path is perfect, and it encourages us to keep trying despite the mistakes and conflicts that are always just waiting to happen. Failed experiences usually stick in the mind. After all, everyone has experienced a low point, but not everyone has experienced success.

PUTTING TOGETHER A BOARD OF CAREER ADVISORS

As we discussed in chapter 10, a board of career advisors is made up of people who serve many purposes and fill many roles, such as mentor, advocate or champion, confidant, role model, and even critic. Members of this board may include colleagues and other acquaintances, members of your professional network, family, and friends. You could meet with each in person, by phone, or online on a regular (daily, weekly, monthly, quarterly) or sporadic basis.

Your board gives you diverse perspectives as well as access to resources and information that you can't get anywhere else. (We're not talking about sharing organizational secrets here; remember, true professionals practice discretion and divulge no confidential or irrelevant work-related information.) This way, it is a huge contributor to your personal and professional growth.

When assembling your board, think of the individuals who come to mind when you ask these questions:

- Who has encouraged my professional development and made me a better leader?
- Who has contributed to my success by guiding and/or advising me?
- Who has challenged me and holds me to my goals?
- Who sees my potential?
- Whom do I admire?
- Whose leadership style (e.g., servant leadership, character-driven leadership) would I like to emulate?
- Who has a strong reputation or personal brand in the industry or community?

Plus, don't overlook your "competitors" or those who are pursuing the same things you're after. Add them to your board as well. They're competition *not* in the true sense of that word (because really you're competing with only yourself and running your career path at your own pace; as we've said in an earlier chapter, you shouldn't compare yourself to others) but in the context of having someone challenge you to get in the game in the first place, to set your bar higher, to hold yourself accountable for the results.

Most important, just like in networking, always consider how you can serve the members of this board and maintain a relationship and rapport with each of them. Popping up in their lives every once in a while and only when you need a favor is never, ever advisable. Make a true effort in this regard.

In case you're wondering what a board of advisors looks like, here's a peek into ours. We wrote our respective lists in first person to give you a flavor of what each member on our board truly means to us.

Laurie's board:

- The pragmatist: Wes, my husband, keeps me grounded when I want to fly away. When I make an assumption, he challenges it with realistic considerations. When I want to jump, he asks me to be more deliberate and weigh the risks.

- The perspective: Natalie, my peer and coauthor, gets me and has invaluable insight into the challenges and circumstances that I face professionally. She understands where I've been and where I'm going, and she inspires me to push harder.

- The cheerleader: Mike always encourages me no matter what. He believes in me and picks me up by the scruff of my neck when I feel broken or when I fall down.

- The professional: Steph is an academic and consultant who is more seasoned than I am career-wise. She is the embodiment of professional development. She has the background (she's "been there") and is very honest and forthcoming about her experiences to help me not only identify any issues or missteps but also reinforce and validate my goals.

- The wise one: Dean is my Yoda, for you *Star Wars* buffs out there. This physician, a longtime client and now friend, is the calm, level-headed voice of reason even amid the most challenging and chaotic of circumstances. He is rational and thorough, patient and composed. His perspective is priceless.

- The catalyst: Eric drives me to be better in my work. If ever I'm inclined to coast, he compels me to push harder. Over the years, we've established a rhythm, spurring strong growth in each other and consistently raising the bar for each other.

- The character builder: Bob is my first mentor. He was very influential and guided me during the early stages of my career. Now, more than a decade later, he continues to be my compass. He demonstrated (and, in turn, shaped in me) those intangibles a leader simply can't put a price on, like integrity and character. His example has had a deep and lasting impact on me.

Natalie's board:

- Rory, my husband, perpetually challenges me and pushes me to learn something new, do something different, demand more from myself, and stretch myself in such a way that I'm always a little uncomfortable and never complacent. As the owner and CEO of several companies, he appreciates what I do as an executive. And, because he is not in healthcare, he offers me perspectives and insights that I don't typically encounter in the industry but have deeply enhanced my strategies.
- Rulon, my fellowship preceptor and later my first healthcare boss, is not only a mentor but also a friend. Because we have known each other since the beginning of my career, I can rely on him to give me well-rounded or global advice that takes into account not just my professional needs and goals but also those of my family and my personal interests. Plus, he is so knowledgeable about the industry that saying he's a great resource is a huge understatement. To put it simply, this man taught me how to be a CEO and to this day inspires me to be the caliber of leader he is. If I'm even half as kind and half as good as he is, I'd consider myself a success.
- Kevin, my mentor and supporter, has been opening his door for me since the first day we met. Not only does he regularly check on my career progress, but he also holds me accountable for the goals I've set for myself. He

never hesitates to ask me the tough questions, does not sugarcoat his opinions, and offers constructive critique of my professional decisions and actions. He's one of the most generous and character-driven people I know, freely giving his time, attention, compassion, and expertise to serve others.

- Laurie, my coauthor and session co-facilitator, needs no introduction. Just as a competitive runner runs better when racing fast runners, I'm encouraged to rise to the occasion and give only my best performance when I'm around such a high achiever and hard worker like Laurie. She and I occupy the same space in our careers, and we each relate to the other's experiences.

- Robb, a colleague and a tireless advocate, is my go-to person for the day-to-day operational issues I encounter in my role. If I'm navigating politically delicate waters, for example, I call him for his advice and input—and he never steers me wrong. The wealth of information, intelligence, lessons, and instincts he eagerly shares with those around him is second only to the warmth, humility, and openness he displays. He is a true servant leader and is a calm and reassuring presence in my life.

- Sheila, a former colleague but a forever friend, is my kindred spirit and cheerleader. She re-energizes me when I'm feeling dejected and overwhelmed, and she doesn't judge me for my shortcomings. She reminds me why I do what I do and why I love it. And she's genuinely happy for my accomplishments and genuinely cares about my well-being—in and out of the office. She also doesn't hesitate to tell me about myself and gives me a proverbial swift kick when needed! We share a bond that transcends backgrounds, experiences, physical distance, busy lives, and everything else.

- Lance, a dear friend, is quirky, kind, and clever. He helps me to self-reflect and make sense of the various dynamics that are constantly in play. He's intellectual and steady.

Perhaps this is why he's a clinical psychologist! He's the listener. The ability to run scenarios by him from several different angles before I encounter them is invaluable.

GETTING STARTED

The first time you meet with a potential mentor, focus on simply having a conversation. Introduce/reintroduce yourself, ask about the person's role and responsibilities, ask follow-up questions about what the person brings up, and listen and watch intently (you can learn a lot about someone just by listening and watching). If personal details enter the discussion, allow them. They're a natural part of a dialogue. Don't (or try not to) ask for a mentoring relationship right out of the gate. After all, you still have to assess whether the person's career path, experience, style, character, and reputation are a good fit with yours (and vice versa). If the initial meeting doesn't turn out to be a mentoring relationship, then at least you've gained another professional to add to your network.

The meeting doesn't have to be face-to-face, which is difficult to do if you and your potential mentor are in two different cities or states. You could talk on the phone or perhaps through Skype. For a high-profile mentor (e.g., a large-system CEO), often you will have to schedule a time to talk or have lunch or dinner, not just pick up the phone to make casual plans.

Serving the Mentor

At the start of (or even before) a new mentoring relationship, you may be plagued with feelings of intimidation, inadequacy, and self-doubt. You may wonder, "What do I have to offer this person?" And you're right on track when you worry about this, because it means you understand the give-and-take nature of mentorship.

Let's repeat what we've said before: You *do* have something to offer. Much of a mentoring relationship is the imparting of wisdom by the mentor to the mentee. But the mentee doesn't come to this union empty-handed. Exhibit 11.1 breaks down the contributions of a mentee.

Doing what you can to serve or give to your mentor (instead of just taking) shows that you're an active participant in the mentoring process. Know what else you can do? Apply what you're learning to your everyday life, try out advice that resonates with you, and make improvements according to the mentor's feedback. Doing this will energize you professionally. Plus, it will show your mentor (and others) that you're serious about and committed to your own development.

Exhibit 11.1 What a Mentee Can Offer to a Mentor

- *Time.* A hospital CEO has precious little time, but you—at this stage in your career—can spare some time and be flexible. So be selfless. When making an appointment with your mentor, accommodate his or her schedule (even if it's after work hours). Show up or call on time and prepare for the meeting, gathering all your questions, concerns, and updates beforehand to make the meeting as productive as possible. And don't go over the time allotted (or worse, monopolize the entire conversation with sporadic questions) because, more often than not, your mentor must get back to a pressing task or project. The point is not only to maximize the time carved out for you but also to be respectful of your mentor's other commitments. Sometimes you may be of help by simply listening to your mentor. Tune into that and identify any areas where you can help out.

- *Connections.* You may think your professional circle pales in comparison to that of your seasoned mentor (and in most ways, it probably does). However, in some ways your circle may be bigger than your mentor's because you're likely more social media savvy. You could help your mentor enlarge or strengthen this network by introducing him or her to online forums and other resources.

- *Resources.* Combined, your time flexibility, Internet savvy, and networking skills put you in a position to solve a problem that your mentor may be grappling with. You could offer to do some online and offline research, to consult with your board of career advisors or

(continued)

peers, or to review proposals or other documents. In this way, your mentor sees you as an extension, another pair of eyes and hands that can help when needed.

- *Expertise*. What's your sweet spot? Are you an expert in a certain area (like coding, blogging, or marketing)? If so, make it known. You may be able to serve as a resource, an informal advisor, or a sounding board to your mentor. If not, hone a skill or gain knowledge in whatever area you're passionate about. It can't hurt you to be an expert just for the sake of serving those who serve you.

GIVING BACK TO THE FIELD

It's never too early to start identifying opportunities to be a mentor. Mentoring others is how you can start giving back to your profession. Every lesson learned, conflict encountered, challenge conquered, failure experienced, or mission accomplished results in dos and don'ts that you can pass on to those who are a few steps behind you. Are you an expert at this point? No. But you don't need to be an expert to warn someone of pitfalls and barriers, to point someone in the right direction, to share your experience, and to answer questions so that others can manage their expectations.

Some young careerists give back by teaching, as we both did (and still do). Natalie, while just starting her career at Poudre Valley, served one semester as an instructor of a leadership and management course for the Institute of Business and Medical Careers. Since then, she has taught for various programs, including the University of New Mexico's Anderson Executive MBA (master of business administration) program and Brigham Young University's Marriott School MHA (master of healthcare administration) program. Likewise, Laurie, at age 25, was invited to teach an undergraduate course in healthcare administration for a semester at Creighton University. She subsequently held faculty appointments at Clarkson College, Methodist College, and Bellevue University in their respective undergraduate and graduate healthcare administration programs. Now, Laurie's teaching career has come full circle with a return to Creighton University as a faculty member, director of healthcare leadership programs, and the program director for Creighton's Executive MBA in Healthcare Management.

Plus, we both are mentors and frequently volunteer as career coaches, resume reviewers, and mock interview partners. Our annual early careerist session at the American College of Healthcare Executives (ACHE) Congress on Healthcare Leadership is another way that we extend a hand to those who will be serving the field in the future.

We've all been at that crossroad, not knowing whether we should turn right or left or go straight as we move along our career path. Be that person who reaches out to hand someone a road map. You don't need to tell the person where to go; you just have to show where he or she is at this point in the journey.

Giving back is a good way for you to practice your leadership skills. You are, after all, among the next generation of healthcare leaders. This is your chance to be a role model, a shining example—to others and to yourself. Be the kind of strong mentor that you've always wanted. Be the kind of leader that you'd be proud to follow.

Rookie Mistakes

Putting People on a Pedestal

One way that you could better relate to those in the top ranks (so that you won't be as intimidated to approach them as mentors) is to *not* put them on a pedestal, no matter how much you admire them. They're only human, after all.

While attending ACHE's Congress many years ago, Laurie attended a lecture given by a highly accomplished hospital executive, whom Laurie saw (and still sees) as a role model

→

and whom she had thus put on a pedestal. This executive shared story after story about her career—from being overlooked for promotions to being "restructured" by her organization to living through major failures to accepting her own shortcomings. As Laurie listened, she began to see not only the similarity between the executive's experiences and her own but also the authenticity (read: ups and downs) of the executive's journey. She also realized that successful leaders are not magical beings who do everything perfectly all the time and who never grapple with mistakes and difficulties. It was an encouraging lecture for Laurie—as well as an eye-opening one.

Assuming a Mentoring Relationship Without Working for It

Don't be that person who assumes that your colleague's or friend's mentor is also your own—simply because you've met, had a few conversations with, or been around that mentor. You must earn a mentee position. It takes a lot more than a meet-and-greet, a five-minute chat or follow-up e-mail, or a casual association to establish a mentoring relationship. Be self-aware enough to know when you're overstepping your bounds. And be respectful of the relationships that your friends and colleagues have worked hard to foster—not for your benefit but for their own.

Remember These

- Mentors see the potential in you, and they do what they can to nudge (even push) you toward becoming the person or professional you could be.

→

- Surround yourself with individuals who don't soothe and coddle your ego all the time. Such a mentor understands that a candid critique will strengthen your character, skills, and performance better than nonstop praise (which may not always be genuine) and agreement can ever do.

- Don't be afraid to ask a CEO or senior executive to be your mentor. They were in your shoes once, so they'll be able to relate to your early career experiences and mentoring needs.

- As a mentee, you can't expect to get helpful advice and guidance from your mentor if you aren't honest about yourself and your concerns, worries, goals, and dreams.

- A board of career advisors is made up of people who serve many purposes and fill many roles, such as mentor, advocate or champion, confidant, role model, and even critic.

- Doing what you can to serve or give to your mentor (instead of just taking) shows that you're an active participant in the mentoring process.

Opening Doors of Opportunity for Yourself

FOR UP-AND-COMERS LIKE you, nothing is as constructive as the wisdom of people who have firsthand experiences with the processes and activities you are now undertaking. Just as you wouldn't take resume-writing tips from someone whose resume is cluttered with long sentences and unnecessary details, you wouldn't listen to healthcare career advice from someone who has never studied or worked in the field or never held the position you aspire to fill. This theme runs throughout this book, but it's especially apparent in part III because this is where you take the critical first steps into healthcare management, so you need guidance from those who have worn the shoes you now walk in, so to speak.

Are you a student amid an internship year or the competitive process of searching and applying for internships? A recent graduate going from job interview to job interview? Or a new hire navigating the ins and outs of your first role in the field? Regardless of where you fall in this early-career spectrum, we have you covered. The advice and insights we offer here (in fact, throughout the book) are not only applicable to your situation today but also useful resources for your younger colleagues or even mentees in the future. That's because we include only suggestions and ideas that are classic or timeless, not trendy. When we urge you in 2018 to take full advantage of the exposure to leadership afforded by your internship, for example, we guarantee that in 2028 we will still be promoting that same message (but, of course, tailored for that future environment). The same goes when we insist today that you prepare well for job (and internship) interviews and that you actively pursue (not passively wait for) career opportunities and personal/professional improvement.

These lessons are the same ones passed on to us by our mentors and the generations of leaders and experts who came before and with us. And now we're sharing them with you in hopes that you will use them not just to get your foot in the door but also to open that door wide for yourself and for others.

Note to My 25-Year-Old Self

At age 25, newly married and serving as an administrative dietitian responsible for a 500-bed hospital kitchen, I knew I needed to complete postgraduate work to advance my career. Little did I know then that my educational journey would lead me beyond dietetics and into healthcare leadership. Working full time and taking healthcare administration classes on a part-time basis opened my eyes, both academically and practically. I had opportunities to network internally and become involved in hospitalwide committees. By age 30, I had transitioned into hospital administration.

A guiding principle early on should be network or no work. Understand the value of connections—in the workplace, in the local community, and in the industry. Your network will serve as the foundation for your career and will be a resource to draw on—from securing a fellowship to job advancement to industry leadership appointment. Developing a strong network of connections does not just happen; it is an investment that needs to be cultivated and maintained.

Take strategic risks. Be creative, and try new things. Accept new challenges, and do not be afraid of change. Never stop learning, and keep adding to your toolbox of job skills. It is so much better to accept roles that interest you or that are aligned with your career goals than to be "volunteered" and then find yourself in a direction you would not have chosen. Do not be afraid to stretch yourself and show others your capabilities. Do your best to stay positive, even if you find yourself busy making lemonade out of the lemons coming your way.

Few people work alone, so when you are building your team, surround yourself with strong people. Choose individuals who complement your strengths and weaknesses and who share your values; you will learn from them, and they will challenge you to perform at your highest potential. Together, you will form a strong, successful team that will outperform anything you could do alone.

Take time to give back to the profession and the community. Mentor or coach others either in your own organization or beyond. Visit student groups or provide shadowing experiences to encourage those entering or advancing in the field. Serve on community committees/boards that interest you and that will benefit from your presence. You will gain new knowledge from those experiences, which will be useful in your career, and you will be enriched by the opportunity to serve.

Never forget the Golden Rule while traveling along your professional path. Your professional reputation and personal brand will thank you.

Lastly, seek out mentors and coaches. Their insights will be invaluable to your success. Take every opportunity to learn from those who have been there and whose wisdom will equip you to grapple with the challenges of leadership.

Remember to take time for yourself and your family. Your organization and your home team will be better off with a happy, healthy person at the helm.

May you do great things—and have some fun along the way as well!

Signed,
Deborah Y. Rasper, LFACHE
Governor (2006–2009), American College of Healthcare Executives
Retired Administrator, St. Vincent Mercy Hospital

CHAPTER 12

Grab That Internship!

The distinction between "assistant" and "intern" is a simple one: assistants are paid, interns are not. But of course interns are paid, in experience.

—*Joyce Carol Oates, novelist*

Reading Points

- How It Works

- Applying for an Internship

- Create Your Own Internship

- The End of an Internship

ADMINISTRATIVE INTERNSHIPS, FELLOWSHIPS, and residencies. These terms can mean different things in different organizations, but for the sake of simplicity and argument, we're going to consider them all one and the same; we'll refer to them as *internship* in this chapter.

An internship is a bridge between your academic and professional paths, between the end of your schooling and the beginning of your career. For that reason, an internship is both educational and experiential. It requires the intern to perform real-world tasks and to apply classroom techniques—such as group discussions, hands-on training, one-on-one coaching, questions and answers, writing a paper, and doing a presentation—to make sense of what has been learned from the internship activities. This is a fantastic setup!

Because an internship exposes you to the highest executive levels, it introduces you to engaging and prominent roles within the organization. It can launch your career, redirect your career path, serve as your fertile learning environment, and assist you in building unprecedented networking relationships. Although often an internship does not materialize into a job, it prepares you for the realities and expectations of the work world—whether your goal as an intern is (1) to prepare yourself to move straight from the classroom to an administrative office or (2) to be groomed as a leader in a specific type of organization.

Among the things you'll gain during an internship are

- meaningful relationships;
- mentors;
- references;
- an understanding of operational, clinical, and financial areas of the organization as well as ancillary and support departments or partners;
- working knowledge of important processes, including strategic planning, financial analysis, budgeting, project management, process design and implementation, change initiatives, and so on;
- insight into physician arrangements, physician specialties, the physician–administrator relationship, and physician referral patterns (which specialties generally consult with other specialties);
- a sense of organizational culture dynamics;

- the ability to speak the language of healthcare—that is, general and specific terms, acronyms, shortcuts and slang, and so on; and
- an understanding of payers (private and public) and payment models.

Among the practical things you'll learn are how to

- run meetings for a department, executives, a project team, and so on;
- collaborate with multiple stakeholders;
- form and lead a team;
- perform analytics;
- create a strategic plan;
- develop, implement, and monitor a process;
- interview job applicants (and, by extension, how to prepare yourself for a job interview);
- spot, correct, and report errors or wrongdoing;
- embrace or support culture;
- create and read a pro forma;
- write a white paper; and
- procure a piece of equipment or service from request for proposal to negotiation to signed contract.

In this chapter, we explain how internships provide invaluable experiences, learning, and connections. We discuss how internship works, how to find one, how to take advantage of its many benefits, and how to create internship opportunities where none exist.

HOW IT WORKS

The structure of an internship can vary from program to program, depending on the culture of the organization, the longevity of the existing program, the vision and direction of the current program preceptor, and so on. Sometimes an internship takes place during the school semester, something that you could incorporate into your class schedule. Sometimes it takes place the semester after you graduate or during summer break. Sometimes it is paid, and other times it is unpaid.

Typically, an internship lasts for only one year, but it can accelerate your career by three to five years (perhaps more).

At the beginning of your internship, you may be handed an outline or a schedule for the year. It may include your expected duties, such as rounding on different departments for a certain amount of time (e.g., one department for one month, four departments for three months each). It also may specify the meetings you're expected to attend and the projects you're expected to complete. At the completion of your internship, you may be required to write a paper or do a formal presentation in front of the program preceptor, organizational leadership, department directors, or other personnel.

The essence of internship is exposure. Count on being introduced to the inner workings of departments and the organization as a whole, the community at large, the movers and shakers inside and outside the organization, myriad change initiatives, bureaucracy and politicking, all levels of personnel, and so much more. Take advantage of all of it.

The harsh reality is that, in one year, your "seat at the table" will end, and you will no longer have an all-access pass to senior management (until, of course, that day when you become part of that team). So while you're serving as intern, gain as much real-world knowledge and experience as you can, maximize your exposure and proximity to experienced leaders, try new things and develop new skills, and look for or create opportunities that can extend your tenure or turn your internship into a full-time position. For example, when Natalie was a fellow at a health system, she was charged with designing the organization's retail strategic plan. When she presented the plan to the board at the end of her fellowship, she impressed them enough that she was hired as the full-time director of retail services.

Tips for Taking Advantage of Your Internship

- *Get to know the role of your preceptor.* Similar to a manager, a preceptor is the person you will report to throughout your intern year. The preceptor answers your questions, helps you gain access where and when you need it, gives you feedback, and guides your every step. You will likely meet with your preceptor regularly—often weekly—so that he or she can check on your progress, keep you on track, brainstorm project ideas, and give advice and direction. Sometimes, a private debriefing with your preceptor is necessary. For example, after you've observed certain occurrences (e.g., critical decision-making moments, community interactions, strategy or policy changes, disagreements), you may ask questions about what happened, why it happened, and whether there's a historical context or precedent to what occurred. This is one of the ways you can learn about the inner workings of the organization.

  Understand that your preceptor is expecting you to have many questions, so don't be shy or afraid to ask away! The preceptor (along with everyone else in the organization) assumes you are sharp, prepared, and thoughtful but not necessarily someone who knows everything. In fact, she or he might think you know less than you actually do given that interns have different backgrounds and varying degrees of experiences and thus know-how. Despite what you know or don't know, the preceptor is expecting that you'll meet your deadlines, produce good work, and ask for clarifications when you are unsure.

  If you gel well with your preceptor, he or she can become a valuable reference during your internship and even a longstanding mentor after your internship. Natalie and her preceptor, for example, have remained good friends for years, and he has proven to be an invaluable mentor, colleague, and friend. She relies on him to offer his perspective and general guidance when she faces tough situations. Because he is genuinely proud of her and views her success as an extension of his own, she shares news of her accomplishments with him and acknowledges and thanks him for his countless and selfless contributions to her growth.

- *Interview a leader from a different department every month.* One is great, but more is better. Take them to lunch or coffee, and pick their brain. Ask them how they got to where they are, what they do, and how their specific role (e.g., overall responsibilities, departmental goals, daily duties) fits into the organization. Such a conversation will give you insight into how the organization operates, part by part and inside out. Plus, it will help you define which service or operational area you'd like to learn more about or specialize in once your program ends.

  Don't forget to ask the leader if you could add him or her to your network. Most important, volunteer to help with projects or tasks in the executive's department if your schedule allows or if your preceptor approves. Volunteering will not only help you initiate a relationship with the leader but also give you the opportunity to learn about her or his area.

  If you sit down with one executive per month, by the end of the year you will have 12 new experts in your network with whom you could build a relationship. Sustain these networking relationships.

  And don't forget the doctors and other clinicians! Approach them, too. Get acquainted with their perspective. How do they view administration? What can leaders do to better serve patients and their families, to involve the clinical side in organizational initiatives, to improve relationships between physicians and the hospital?

- *Keep an internship journal.* Jot down your daily activities, key learning moments, progress made on your projects, tidbits of information, and pearls of wisdom. You might find that you'll reference this record for years to come!

- *Dive into as many organizational areas as possible.* If your internship plan doesn't include a department or unit, specialty, service line, program, or initiative you'd like to get involved in and learn about, ask your preceptor if it could be added. The organization likely will allow you to go for whatever piques your interest. In fact, some internship programs give interns carte blanche or full access to almost every part of the organization, enabling interns to observe and even participate in the activities or projects of the units. If this is the case, ask to be assigned to every conceivable area possible. You could be a member of the performance improvement team, sit in on governing board meetings, shadow an emergency room manager during a full shift, or assist the chief operating officer and her staff with the implementation of a new policy.

     By diving in, you can whittle down the list of the areas you do and do not want to work in once you become a practicing healthcare manager. For example, if you spent an internship month working on quality improvement projects and tasks and absolutely hated that kind of detailed work, now you know not to pursue a position that heavily relies on that skill set. Again, self-awareness is critical at this point. If you understand your strengths and weaknesses, you can better steer the direction of your career path.

There is no better time than during an internship to immerse yourself in myriad experiences, determine what you like and don't like about a particular area or the world of healthcare in general, learn a lot and from the best, and ask for guidance and feedback.

Internship is also the time to hone your interpersonal, listening, and critical thinking skills and to practice your ability to follow directions, execute plans, and try new things or take risks.

APPLYING FOR AN INTERNSHIP

The rigors and prestige of many internship programs make acceptance into these programs highly selective. Plus, there are always more student candidates than internship positions, so open spots are tough to find. If you are facing this dilemma, apply to multiple internship programs; if you're willing, apply to those that are out of your immediate area.

1. *Application form.* The form is usually lengthy, so be patient and fill it out completely and accurately. Natalie has been on selection panels and has witnessed entire applications thrown out because of minor spelling errors or incomplete sections. Because they receive so many applications, most selection committees are not shy about pitching those that are less than perfect. Take your time when filling out this application, have someone else proofread your work, and send out only your best effort.

2. *Essay.* It's totally appropriate to ask someone who is further along in his or her career (like a mentor or an older colleague) to look over your essay—not just for grammar or syntax but also for overall content. How well does your essay reflect real-world expectations and healthcare realities? Does it make sense in the current healthcare environment? If you are still a student, your experience in the real-world trenches is limited, so allow your experienced colleague to guide you. Your essay will invariably be stronger after you make the edits suggested by your colleague.

    Tap into your network or board of career advisors and invite some of them to speak with you candidly about your strengths and weaknesses as well as your chances of landing available internship opportunities. Use their feedback to answer essay questions such as, What do you hope to get out of this internship?

Often, applications include one general essay question or a series of three or four questions. Give each one the attention it deserves. You may use key terms—such as *commitment, self-discipline, tenacity* or *perseverance, character, experience, learning orientation, service,* and *meaningful or valuable work*—to bolster your arguments. If needed, dig into your old high school guidebooks about how to structure sentences, paragraphs, and essays. Selection panels assess application essays on their grammar and syntax as much as on their content. Keep in mind that a well-thought-out essay can be used from application to application, with only slight modifications (tailored to fit the organization's internship requirements).

3. *References.* Choose your references wisely! Ask people who (1) have seen your work and know your potential to perform at high levels if given a great opportunity and (2) will speak well about your skills and knowledge as well as your character. Some internship programs require that you submit a letter of reference, while others ask that you provide the contact information for your references so that the programs can call your references directly. Either way, get permission from your references and give them a heads-up that they might be contacted. No one wants to be surprised or caught unprepared to vouch for you. Lastly, before you furnish a list of references, make sure that the people on the list are still alive, still willing to give you a reference, and still can be reached at their listed phone number. A fantastic reference with out-of-date contact information isn't worth a thing and is embarrassing!

4. *Interview.* There are so many candidates for internships that a phone interview will almost always be done first to weed out the competition. A face-to-face interview will follow. (See chapter 13 for more discussion on interviewing; some of our suggested strategies in that chapter— especially how you present yourself and interact with the interviewers—apply to internship interviews as well.)

Final thoughts on applying for internships: Apply early and apply often. Internships are cyclical and usually run from July to July; they may be awarded as far in advance as the beginning of the calendar year. It's prudent to start looking for internships for the following year just after summer of the preceding year. Application due dates vary from program to program. If you are applying to many (which you should be doing), create a spreadsheet to track the process and due dates for each program.

Lean on Your School Network to Find Internship Opportunities

Talk to the director of your health administration program to find out if he or she knows of alumni whom you could approach for an internship opportunity; it's a bonus if they work for an organization in which you want to intern. Ask second-year students where they interned their first year. Ask recent graduates where they interned while in school. Contact your network, board of career advisors (if any), professors, and classmates for suggestions. Once word spreads that you are seeking guidance, opportunities or leads may come your way. (As we've mentioned in earlier chapters, we don't advise you to get in touch with your networking contacts only to ask them for a favor. Reach out to them only after you've already built rapport; otherwise, they'll feel used and will disengage from your network.)

You may check out these resources as well:

- The alumni association of your college or university
- State chapters of associations, like the American College of Healthcare Executives, Medical Group Management Association, and Healthcare Financial Management Association
- Local or national health systems' online job boards
- The career section of the website of trade organizations and healthcare associations
- State hospital associations' careerist resources
- Human resources departments

CREATE YOUR OWN INTERNSHIP

If you can't move across the country or to a different town for a few months of internship, or if you can't spend an entire semester getting paid nothing or next to nothing, you can still make an internship work for you and your unique situation. How? Walk into the human resources department of the hospital or healthcare organization you would like to be a part of, and ask about an internship. It's an uncommon and bold move, but it can pay off.

When Laurie was completing her master's degree in healthcare administration, her program hosted a visiting lecturer one evening—the CEO of a local health system. Several months later, as she approached the final semester of her program, she cold-called the CEO to inquire about internship opportunities. He offered her a semester-long, part-time internship. If the story stopped here, it would be good enough, but it got better. Halfway through that internship, the vice president of clinic operations was terminated. Laurie, who was aware she was very light on qualifications for this big role, asked the CEO if she could apply for the position anyway. He took a chance and gave her the nod (remember this story from chapter 9?). She became the next vice president of clinic operations for the organization—thanks to the internship that brought her there.

If you don't have the time to participate in an in-person internship, you could still pursue a learning opportunity by first contacting the director of human resources for the organization you want to serve. Ask to interview the director for one hour about the areas you're interested in. Select an area based on the information you obtained, and then develop a working relationship with the head of that area. Volunteer your free services for a certain amount of time (e.g., one hour once a week for three months). For example: "I would love an internship, but I have a full-time job. But I'd like a chance to work with you on a project. I'm available a few hours a week for the next few months. I can work for free." What organization would turn down this offer?

If this approach doesn't work, you could at least forge networking relationships and add the organization as a reference.

Job Shadowing

A casual, but no less valuable, way to garner real-world experience is job shadowing. Obtained through the same methods as landing an internship, job shadowing entails following a professional for a few hours or a few days as he or she performs daily duties. This is a great way to get your foot in the door to future internship and full-time positions as well as to meet people you could add to your network. If you shadow someone once per semester throughout your two-year graduate program, by the time you finish school you'll have gained four new experiences and four new networking contacts. That's a huge payoff for a small investment of time!

THE END OF AN INTERNSHIP

All good things come to an end. Because most internships do not lead to permanent positions, you must develop a plan for the next adventure in your career. About four to six months before you complete your internship, begin your job hunt. For example, Natalie approached her internship very strategically. About six months into it, she started looking and applying for jobs. This way, she thought, her transition from internship to employment would be seamless and she would be gainfully employed by a healthcare organization by the time her fellowship was over. Luckily, her internship led to a position in the same organization (see her earlier story of how she became the director of retail services).

If you like the organization where you are interning, speak to your preceptor or someone else about any potential fits for your skill set. If no positions are available or will open up in the near future, look elsewhere. You know that network that you've worked so hard to build up and maintain? Now is the time to use it. Ask for appropriate references, update your resume (add all the awesome things you did during your internship), scan the job ads, and fill out applications. Good luck!

Remember These

- An internship prepares you for the realities and expectations of the work world—whether your goal as an intern is (1) to prepare yourself to move straight from the classroom to an administrative office or (2) to be groomed as a leader in a specific type of organization.

- While you're serving as intern, gain as much real-world knowledge and experience as you can, maximize your exposure and proximity to experienced leaders, try new

→

---

things and develop new skills, and look for or create opportunities that can extend your tenure or turn your internship into a full-time position.

- Understand that your preceptor is expecting you to have many questions, so don't be shy or afraid to ask away! The preceptor (along with everyone else in the organization) assumes you are sharp, prepared, and thoughtful but not necessarily someone who knows everything.

- By diving into as many organizational areas as possible, you can whittle down the list of the areas you do and do not want to work in once you become a practicing healthcare manager.

- The rigors and prestige of many internship programs make acceptance into these programs highly selective. Plus, there are always more student candidates than internship positions, so open spots are tough to find.

- Take your time when filling out an internship application, have someone else proofread your work, and send out only your best effort. A slight mistake or an incomplete form could hurt your chances.

- Because most internships do not lead to permanent positions, you must develop a plan for the next adventure in your career. About four to six months before you complete your internship, begin your job hunt.

CHAPTER 13

Master the Job Interview

Be so good they can't ignore you.

—*Steve Martin, actor*

Reading Points

- The Preparation Stage
- The Interview Stage
- The Follow-Up Stage
- Salary and Benefits Negotiation

THE MOST COMMONLY asked questions we receive from new health administration graduates who attend our American College of Healthcare Executives Congress on Healthcare Leadership seminar revolve around the job interview. It makes sense. After all, you can't start a career path until you land a job. And you can't land a job if you don't ace that interview. Plus, often you can't move on to another organization or apply for a bigger and better position without going through the interview process. To a careerist, the interview is as inevitable and as life-changing as failure.

By the time you sit for the interview—the face-to-face, question-and-answer, resume explanation portion of the process—you should already have done a lot of legwork to present yourself in the best light. That's because the interview is merely one stage, sandwiched between the preparation and the follow-up stages. Successful interviewees know that this much work goes into the process. Therefore, they master all components of each stage, leaving nothing to chance.

Preparation. Interview. Follow-up. Let's dig into each of them in this chapter.

THE PREPARATION STAGE

Just as you shouldn't show up to a certification exam without having studied, you shouldn't show up to a job interview without having prepared. Preparation is a must to ensure that, during the interview, you can respond thoughtfully to questions, feel and look professional but at ease, articulate relevant job experiences and qualifications, pose informed questions, and ultimately convince the interview panel that you are the right person for the position.

At the prep stage, gather as much information as you can—not just on the job qualifications and responsibilities but also on the organization and the interviewers. Take copious notes. Review those notes over and over. Memorize details if you can.

Research the Organization

During an interview, nothing is worse than being clueless about the organization you're interviewing with. From the organization's perspective, you don't care enough about becoming a member of its team because you didn't even bother to get to know it. From the interviewer's perspective, you are wasting everybody's time.

Don't leave that impression. That's as bad as a no-call, no-show, which burns bridges.

So what should you know? Learn the organization's mission, vision, and values. Relate them to your own beliefs as you study. In the past ten years, neither of us remembers a time when the interviewer didn't ask, Which one of our values resonated with you the most? Know how to answer that and similar questions.

Familiarize yourself with the history, type of services, awards, patient mix, and locations of the organization. Has the hospital been a part of the community since 1940, or did it just open five years ago after separating from a regional system? Is it an acute care, a specialty care, or an outpatient facility; a for-profit or not-for-profit? Does it have a Level I trauma center, a neonatal intensive care unit, a cancer center? What awards or recognitions has it earned lately? What system is it affiliated with? Is it freestanding? When you know these details, you can better weigh job-related decisions, such as transfer opportunities—that is, if you're open to moving to other locations within the larger organization.

Start your research with the company's website, and then branch out from there to industry publications and even Google searches (using the organization's name as well as its top leadership). Check its social media pages, which document its current news and events as well as showcase its overall culture and personality. Ask your networking contacts if they know any current or past employees of the organization. Tap your former undergraduate or graduate school classmates to see whether anyone has interned or worked there.

Take the time to do your research, and do it well. (Natalie, for example, gives herself five to seven days to properly prepare for an interview.) The knowledge (or lack of knowledge) you bring to the interview speaks volumes about you and your intention to secure a second interview and ultimately a job. We argue that this preparation is just as (if not more) important as your performance during the actual interview.

Research the Interview Panel

Whether your interview panel consists of one or ten people, educate yourself about them. Doing so shows that you are interested in and care about these individuals (not to mention the job itself), are personable, and are professional. Furthermore, it allies you to the interviewers and generally makes you approachable and memorable. Two good sources of this information are the organization's online staff directory (if you can access it) and LinkedIn (many professionals have profiles). Google also works.

Learn each panelist's name, title or role, responsibilities, and background. Background information serves as conversation fodder, which helps you create an instant connection with panelists. For example, you may find that an interviewer went to the same school, came from the same state, or volunteers for the same charitable cause as you. You can use this common ground to strike up a conversation or break the ice. When interviewers can relate to you, they can picture themselves working with you.

Remembering people's names is invaluable in any situation, but more so during an interview. Address interviewers by name when you respond, such as "Well, Mary, I'm glad you asked that question!" or "Thanks, Bob, I agree with that philosophy." This makes the interview less impersonal and more intimate. Natalie once interviewed with a ten-person panel. Because she did her research on each person and matched each face with his or her name, she knew everyone even before they introduced themselves. She tacked on the interviewer's name to her answers, something that wowed the panel because, in their view, she had just learned their name. It was a savvy move that convinced them she has a quick mind that absorbs a lot of information even in a stressful situation. That gave her an edge over the other applicants. And guess what? She got the job.

Practice Your Elevator Speech

An elevator speech is a brief (about 30 to 60 seconds or long enough to deliver during an elevator ride) description of who you are, what you do, what you're passionate about, what you want to accomplish, and other details specific to your career path. It's a high-level summary of your personal brand. It should include your career goals and aspirations. That's a lot of important stuff to fit into less than a minute! But sometimes those seconds feel like forever when you don't know what else to say.

Your elevator speech shouldn't be a regurgitation of your resume. Boring. The interviewers have your resume in front of them, so there's no need to repeat the information. Share something about your passion and experiences, something that's not included or hard to explain on a resume. But limit the personal details you include—no pet names, favorite color, or silly or irrelevant information. Here's a sample elevator speech: "I'm a Tennessee native who is passionate about leadership development, clinical quality improvement, and collaborating with healthcare practitioners to maximize efficiency in patient care processes. My studies and internship experiences show that I thrive in small organizations and communities, where I can readily observe the impact of my efforts and build meaningful relationships with fellow employees and local stakeholders." None of this appears on a resume, and no non-work-related details are included.

The first question just about every interviewer poses is, Tell me a little about yourself. If you come prepared to deliver a well-written and well-practiced elevator speech, you can relax when you hear this question. That calm and in-control demeanor then sets the tone for the rest of your interview. You're already batting a thousand! You've got the first question right! Nice start; it builds your confidence.

Conduct a Mock Interview

"Practice makes perfect" applies to shooting free throws and playing the piano just as much as it does to interviewing. Start holding mock interviews at least five days in advance of your interview. Here are guidelines for doing it right:

1. *Recruit a reliable, serious partner to play the interviewer role.* This person may be a family member, friend, mentor, or member of your board of career advisors. Make sure he or she takes this exercise seriously and won't break character at any time during the interview. To add to the person's authenticity, ask him or her to wear business attire.

2. *Set some rules.* No joking around. No time-outs. No do-overs or mulligans. No getting up to answer the phone or the door or a text or an e-mail; in fact, set aside a whole hour without distractions. That goes for your mock interviewer as well. Tell everyone you have an appointment so that they don't visit or call/text. The only effective way to practice is to treat the process as real.

3. *Use real-world interview questions.* Have your mock interviewer ask questions taken from your own interview experiences, from a friend or colleague who recently had a big interview, from human resources (HR) departments, and so on. These questions probe your job qualifications; skills, knowledge, and abilities; specific past and current experiences; character traits; leadership style or approaches; attitude about various things; strengths and weaknesses; and so on.

    Here's how you can collect real-world questions, a strategy that has worked for Natalie: The moment you walk out of an interview, immediately jot down as many of the questions you were asked as you can while they are still fresh in your head. In addition, you can call the HR department of any organization to inquire if you can obtain a list of general interview questions. You may also ask friends who recently had interviews for the questions they were asked. Create a personal list or database to organize your collection for future reference. You'll find that the questions are similar from one organization to the next.

Think of unexpected questions as well, and formulate answers for them. This way, you can show the real interviewer how well you've prepared; it may also help you get unstuck if you encounter a difficult question during the actual interview.

4. *Practice your recovery.* Flubbing an answer is likely during an interview. It is a stressful situation, and you're expected to be "on" the whole time. A mock interview is the best time to practice saving yourself from misspeaking, giving wrong or conflicting information, not answering satisfactorily, getting stuck on a question, or making other errors. Learn how to listen to yourself and quickly pick up on your flubs so that you can get back on track. Learn how to pause methodically to collect your thoughts before you speak.

5. *Dress the part.* You don't have to don a skirt/pantsuit or a suit and tie, but we urge you to do so. Dressing professionally puts you in the interviewing frame of mind. At this time, you can break in the new outfit or shoes you bought for the interview.

6. *Practice modulating the speed, volume, cadence, and tone of your voice.* You might have a fabulous answer to every interview question, but if you talk too fast, too loud, or too soft; lower or raise your voice for no reason; or mumble and garble your words, your interviewer won't understand what you're saying (let alone hear your brilliance). Practice speaking slowly, enunciating, and using an upbeat tone. Speaking this way demonstrates

your confidence, interest, and sense of comfort. We've never met a person who didn't speak too fast when nervous or too soft when lacking confidence.

7. *Ask your mock interviewer for feedback afterward.* The important thing to remember is to act on the feedback immediately. For example, if the feedback is "you beat around the bush too much" or "you talk so loud," give more direct responses and adjust your volume at your next mock interview.

THE INTERVIEW STAGE

The day has arrived: interview day. Don't be nervous! OK, maybe being a little nervous is a good thing; it means you care. Because you care, you must pay attention to every detail. Assuming you've prepared properly, the only thing standing between you and a great interview are the details. (Note that the following discussion is geared toward face-to-face interviews, as that's the most common form, but we touch on phone interviews at the end of this section.)

- *Dress professionally but comfortably.* This seems contradictory, but hear us out. If you bought new shoes and clothes, cut off the tags and break them in a few days before the big day. Don't wait until the day to find out that your shoes are too narrow or your shirt is too scratchy. An uncomfortable outfit will only distract you from bringing your A game and hurt your chance to shine.

- *Bring a notebook or padfolio, pens, extra copies of your resume, and business cards if you have them.* The notebook or padfolio and business cards must be free of dirt, doodles and scribbles, stickers, and anything else that makes them look unclean. Copies of your resume must be unwrinkled and crisp. Take notes during the interview, because it shows you're paying attention and keeping up with the flow of information.

- *Carry your things in an organized manner.* That might sound like insignificant, micromanaging advice, but we assure you it matters. Picture yourself walking into the interview room while fumbling with your belongings. Your purse, briefcase, or manbag is slung haphazardly on your shoulder; your notebook or pad and pens and resumes and business cards bulge from one of your hands; your cell phone (which you should tuck in your bag or leave in your car) and coffee cup and keys or coat threaten to jump out of the other hand. You attempt to walk across the room while juggling all these things, hoping nothing falls. Then you dump everything on the desk or table. Finally, you try to straighten yourself out. You do all this before you even shake hands with the interviewer. That's not a very graceful first impression, is it?

- *Smile!* Smile from entrance to exit. Smile at the receptionists, the security guards, the people you encounter in the elevators and hallways, the person who calls you into the interview room, the interviewers, the other candidates, and everyone else in between. A smile brightens your face and puts everyone in a good mood. Most important, it shows you're glad to be there, ready to engage, and thankful for the opportunity.

- *Beware of your body language.* Shake hands firmly and look people directly in the eye, because that shows professionalism and willingness to engage. Watch your mannerisms (e.g., flailing arms, blinking too much) as you speak, because they could distract your audience. Other distractions include yawning, stretching, slouching, laughing or talking too loud, looking around the room instead of at the speaker, and having a blank expression on your face.

- *Use your mock interview experience as a jumping-off point for your responses.* If you properly practiced and did so enough times, no questions (even the unexpected or on the fly) should faze you. Sometimes your practice questions match the actual questions, but often they are different. You should be able to use answers from your mock interviews as a frame of reference for actual questions, such as, Is there anything about you that we haven't talked about that you'd like me to know?

  If you get stuck on a question, take a moment to gain your composure. Restate the question aloud and speak slowly, pausing or using fillers if you need to buy time. "That's a great question, Mark, give me a second to think about that. [Pause] I would say that. . . [Pause]." This might give you five or ten extra seconds, and the interviewer will see your gears are in motion, thinking of the appropriate response. That's OK; no one should penalize you for thinking things through. But don't take too long, as your interview doesn't last forever. Often, the answers come once you start speaking. Again, rely on your extensive preparation. Take a deep breath; you've got this.

- *Ask follow-up and wrap-up questions.* Interviewers usually give you a chance to ask questions. Interviews are as much an opportunity for the organization to get to know you as for you to get to know the organization, its people, and the open position. Always prepare two to three well-thought-out questions to ask when it's your turn (at the end). You could ask job-specific questions that were not covered earlier or that you wanted to clarify. You could ask general questions about aspects of the organization you found interesting while doing your research. You could inquire about the culture, the leadership's vision for the future, the organization's community involvement, and so on. Always keep a pad and pen with you when preparing for an interview. You never know, a question about the organization may pop into your head while you're grocery shopping or eating dinner with friends.

Embrace the chance to turn the tables for a few minutes. It will show you took the initiative to do some research, you're interested and curious, and you're engaged. Natalie, who has interviewed many applicants, rarely hires someone who didn't pose any wrap-up questions. Why? Because not having questions is the quickest way to communicate that you don't care what the organization does and believes in, that you're there to earn a paycheck and do nothing else. (See exhibit 13.1 for examples of questions to ask.)

- *Seek common ground.* As we mentioned earlier, you and the interviewer could find a commonality that builds instant rapport that, in turn, changes the one-sided interview into a friendly, less intimidating conversation ("I see that you sit on the Big Brothers Big Sisters board here in Atlanta, Susan. I had a little sister during my four years of undergrad! It was such an amazing learning experience for me."). Find that common ground and sustain that connection. Not only will it make the interview fun (or at least not dry) and memorable for both of you, but it will help the interviewer envision you as part of his or her team. You know you are nailing the interview when the interviewer is talking as much as you are!

- *Showcase your personal brand.* More than ever, organizations are hiring for fit—not just in terms of skill and aptitude but also in terms of interests and attitudes. If you share and showcase your brand during the interview (through your elevator speech, demeanor, and interaction), you boost your chances of being a top contender for the job.

Exhibit 13.1 Sample Wrap-Up Questions

- What would my first 30 to 60 days look like in this role?
- What attributes are most valuable to succeeding in this role?
- What type of manager do you consider yourself?
- What are the current strategic goals of the organization? What about for your team/department?
- What three words would you use to describe the organization's culture?

Phone Interviews

When you think of the interview process, think of its three ascending levels. First is the resume. You send your resume and cover letter, which are then scanned and passed on to several decision makers, one of whom calls you. The resume level is critical because if you don't look good on paper, you won't advance to the next level. Simple as that. Make sure your resume makes an impact on screeners by being descriptive but streamlined, easy to read and follow (use bullet points and reverse chronological order), and reflective of your personal brand (Giang 2013).

Second is the phone interview. This gatekeeper level screens you and other candidates and decides whether you can proceed to the next stage. Third is the face-to-face interview, which is the ultimate level.

The phone interview is an important step toward a job offer. It's rare for an organization to skip this level—that is, spend time and resources interviewing someone face-to-face simply from an initial scan of a resume. So prepare as much for a phone interview as you would for a face-to-face.

During a phone interview, dress to impress and smile even if the interviewer can't see you. Like we said, act *as if* and let the interviewer hear you smile. When you smile, you will feel great. And that will transmit through the wires. Address the interviewer by name and strive to find a common ground to establish a quick connection. You don't have to watch your body language, but you do have to modulate your voice and speak clearly. Take notes, as these will help you come up with follow-up questions.

Hold the interview in a quiet space. Use a landline, if you can, as cell reception is often unreliable or spotty; you don't want to get cut off in the middle of the interview or to hear static. Block off the interview time and notify others who share the same space (including your roommate, significant other, toddler's babysitter, parents, or coworkers) to prevent sudden noises. Treat the phone interview with the utmost respect and professionalism, as you would a face-to-face interview.

One of the benefits of a phone interview is that if you need to compose yourself or think of an answer, you could ask for a question repeat. "I'm sorry, Arthur, I didn't hear the question. Would you mind repeating it?" This could grant you the extra seconds you need to gather your thoughts.

THE FOLLOW-UP STAGE

Salespeople often say that the fortune is in the follow-up. In the world of healthcare leadership, the fortune and the prestige of landing that new role rely heavily on the follow-up.

Timing is everything here. A handwritten note three weeks after the interview is just about pointless. But a handwritten note that arrives within 24 hours or an e-mail sent within one hour after the interview can be gold. If a same-day note is humanly possible, do it. That or a next-day note will make a positive impression on those you spoke to.

Follow up on every interview, every time. Always have a note card and envelope ready, already addressed and stamped. Write the note and drop it in the mailbox on your way home. See exhibit 13.2 for a sample follow-up note.

Exhibit 13.2 Sample Follow-Up Note

Dear Ms. Winston,

Thank you for the opportunity to interview for the role of Operations Coordinator for Radiation Oncology. It was a pleasure meeting you and your team and learning more about your organization. After touring the department and meeting a few of your staff, I feel confident that I can contribute to your goals for growth in the coming year. I am looking forward to hearing from you soon, and I would be honored to be a part of the ABC Health System team.

Cordially,

Natalie

Likewise, send a follow-up note even if you didn't get the job. Differentiate yourself from the crowd by sending a handwritten note or an e-mail to each panelist upon hearing that you are now out of the running. Convey your gratitude for the opportunity to be considered, and wish each one well in their future endeavors. Such a gracious follow-up makes an impact and communicates the strength of your character. It will remind the panelists of who you are and leave the door open for conversations or roles that might come up down the road.

Networking and interviewing overlap in so many ways, and this is one of them. Even if the interview does not end in a job offer, it may lead to you gaining new network contacts—especially after the note you sent to each panelist. For example, Natalie interviewed at the Mayo Clinic but didn't end up getting the job, although she thought the interview went really well. It turned out she was right; she ended up being considered second to a woman with a PhD who was on sabbatical from the Mayo Clinic. As soon as Natalie heard the news, she mailed a follow-up note to the panelists, thanking each of them for their kindness and the opportunity to interview as well as acknowledging how much she enjoyed the process. She was able to turn that experience into a networking relationship with the same people who interviewed her. What's more, she gained additional great interview experience.

Remember, this is a small industry. Your goodwill and kindness spread, but so does your apathy.

SALARY AND BENEFITS NEGOTIATION

A 2017 survey found that 56 percent of the full-time employees who responded to the survey never negotiated their initial job offer. Of those who did negotiate, older professional workers (aged 35 or older) tended to do it more than their younger counterparts (aged 18 to 34) did (CareerBuilder 2017). Time to change this pattern, folks!

First, do you know that negotiation is an option? Almost always, except in cases where the salary and benefits are fixed (like jobs in the public sector, including the military). Second, do you think it's a waste of time? Never. Don't be bashful when it comes to your livelihood or your worth. You're not being overly aggressive if you demand fair pay and benefits for your hard work, experience, and qualifications. In fact, the same survey said that 45 percent of the companies that participated were open to first-offer negotiations. Educate yourself. Research the market and your industry to find average compensation or level/job-specific wages. Be aware that organizations almost always extend an initial offer that is less than the highest amount they are willing to pay. So go ahead, talk money! Take Laurie's example when she made her own case—twice.

In her first leadership role after graduate school, Laurie negotiated 20 percent more than her initial offer. Her justifications for the higher salary included her master's degree, which wasn't a requirement of the position; her recent experience in a four-month internship within the organization, where she completed a full assessment of the clinic's network; and her knowledge of clinic operations, which eliminated the need to train her.

In another role, Laurie negotiated a higher base compensation as well as an allocation of personal days to invest in maintaining an active presence on the speaking circuit. This not only afforded her the opportunity to flex her entrepreneurial muscle (through continuing to accept select speaking and leadership development engagements) but also boosted the credibility and visibility of her employer.

So when's the time to negotiate? *Not* during the first interview. In fact, don't even bring up compensation at that point because you would come across as someone who's just in it for the money! Do it *after* the organization makes you an offer. You do not have to respond immediately. Go home and do some research (if you haven't already) on market wages and benefits for your job title, level or grade, skills and other qualifications, and job responsibilities—within and outside your industry, profession, and even state. Members of your network may have already given you clues on what ballpark figure to expect, but you want to be armed with solid, market-based information (not hearsay) when you negotiate. Whatever salary and benefits (or perks) you decide to counter the initial offer with, make sure they are not so unreasonable or beyond expectations that the negotiation becomes hostile or uncompromising. Keep the dialogue civil and open.

Make a list of your justifications for the increase. What extra qualifications and training do you have? What unique value are you adding to the position and the department? Tie your request to only objective reasons (e.g., "I have extensive experience, an advanced degree, and certifications") and never to subjective criteria (e.g., "I want my spouse to be able to stay home" or "I need a new car"). If your new employer's response to a raise is no, ask if any other nonsalary concessions can be extended to you. These may include a professional development stipend, relocation expense reimbursement, additional personal or vacation days, or partial flex or telecommuting arrangements.

Bottom line: Be prepared to negotiate by doing your research and writing down your justifications—and make your counteroffer within the time frame given (usually a few days). Know your worth, even if you're just starting out.

Remember These

- The interview is merely one stage, sandwiched between the preparation and the follow-up stages.

- Preparation is a must to ensure that, during the interview, you can respond thoughtfully to questions, feel and look professional but at ease, articulate relevant job experiences and qualifications, pose informed questions, and ultimately convince the interview panel that you are the right person for the position.

- Take the time to do your research, and do it well. The knowledge (or lack of knowledge) you bring to the interview speaks volumes about you and your intention to secure a second interview and ultimately a job.

- Address interviewers by name when you respond. This makes the interview less impersonal and more intimate.

- An elevator speech is a brief description of who you are, what you do, what you're passionate about, what you want to accomplish, and other details specific to your career path.

- Hold mock interviews at least five days in advance of your interview.

- Think of the interview process in terms of its three ascending levels: (1) resume level, (2) phone interview level, and (3) face-to-face interview level.

- Timing is everything in follow-up. A handwritten note three weeks after the interview is just about pointless. But a handwritten note that arrives within 24 hours or an e-mail sent within one hour after the interview can be gold.

- Networking and interviewing overlap in many ways. Even if the interview does not end in a job offer, it may lead to you gaining new network contacts.

- Don't be bashful when it comes to your livelihood or your worth. You're not being overly aggressive if

→

> you demand fair pay and benefits for your hard work, experience, and qualifications.
>
> - Don't negotiate your salary and benefits during the first interview. Do it *after* the organization makes you an offer.

REFERENCES

CareerBuilder. 2017. "More Than Half of Workers Do Not Negotiate Job Offers." Published October 27. http://press.careerbuilder.com/2017-10-27-More-Than -Half-of-Workers-Do-Not-Negotiate-Job-Offers-According-to-New-Career- Builder-Survey.

Giang, V. 2013. "19 Reasons Why This Is an Excellent Resume." *Business Insider.* Pub- lished November 7. www.businessinsider.com/why-this-is-an-excellent-resume -2013-11.

ADDITIONAL RESOURCES

Forbes Coaches Council. 2017. "Succeeding Where Others Fail: 12 Approaches to Handling Panel Interviews." *Forbes Community Voice.* Published November 17. www.forbes.com/sites/forbescoachescouncil/2017/11/17/succeeding-where -others-fail-12-approaches-to-handling-panel-interviews/#5e7d3a067f91.

Kachroo-Levine, M. 2017. "How to Negotiate Salary for Your First Full-Time Job." *Forbes.* Published August 29. www.forbes.com/sites/mayakachroolevine/2017 /08/29/how-to-negotiate-salary-for-your-first-full-time-job/#25dbbb80668f.

Ryan, L. 2017. "How to Answer Ten Common Interview Questions—with Confidence." *Forbes.* Published December 9. www.forbes.com/sites/lizryan/2017/12/09/how -to-answer-ten-common-interview-questions-with-confidence/#6af7bb2a3ef1.

CHAPTER 14

90 Days of Onboarding

You don't have to be great to start, but you have
to start to be great.

—*Zig Ziglar, author and motivational speaker*

Reading Points

- Culture and Components
- Operational Orientation
- Personnel Orientation
- Learn from Those Around You
- Personal Considerations for a New Job
- Winning Early
- Gaining Competency
- The Burden of Youth
- Common Pitfalls to Avoid

CONGRATULATIONS! YOU'VE WORKED hard. You prepared
for your interview, wowed the interviewers, and got the job. Now

the real work begins. You have only one chance to make a first impression, and as a young new leader, it's important that you get it right. It will set the tone for your performance in this role, be instrumental in shaping the type of leader you are, and establish others' impressions and expectations of you.

Making mistakes in the first 90 days can be much more harmful than making the same mistakes 6 or 12 months into the job.

Conversely, getting it right will have a bigger effect in the first 90 days. Think of those first critical days as building the foundation of your identity in this new role. Go into the office every day fully aware that your actions are being followed by your superiors, peers, and, most important, the people you may have been hired to lead.

CULTURE AND COMPONENTS

There is much to learn in any new job, and most of it is not and cannot be taught in schools. You will encounter a steep learning curve. The best way to learn how to navigate your new organization is to observe, listen, and take notes. Every organization is different, so pay attention and adapt; it will make your transition far more successful.

Now you have the opportunity to see how the organization's mission, vision, and values are really lived and how they play out in its culture. You considered these when you vetted the organization during the interview process, and hopefully they resonated with you. The mission, vision, and values can signal how (and in what spirit) the organization is led and what is important to its leaders.

Before your fresh perspective as a newcomer fades, leverage that lens to observe and become familiar with the culture. Look for ways the mission, vision, and values are demonstrated in the everyday workings of the business. Get to know the strategic priorities and key internal and external initiatives that contribute to them, both culturally and operationally. Vetting and establishing your personal fit with the organization is a key step in your assimilation process. After you've completed this step, you'll be in an excellent position to contribute and thrive.

Start organizing your thoughts and observations about the organization, the people you meet, and the information you learn. Be intentional and disciplined in this process. Consider starting a journal of things learned, things to do, and perhaps even things to stop doing. Record this information in any format that works for you. Define a process to revisit this action plan to measure your progress, or even to understand your lack of progress.

OPERATIONAL ORIENTATION

Once you're able to, start looking into the applications, software, and systems that you will be using on a regular basis—finance and payroll systems, databases, performance management software, and the like. Learn how to navigate them so you can quickly become proficient. Dedicate a few minutes every day to the task. Ask for training or orientation. Your naïveté will be understood (and expected) early on, but not so much a few months down the road.

Research files and documents related to your role, as well as all the committees or consortia you'll be asked to serve on. This research will help you learn the lay of the land and ascertain where your predecessor, team, department, and organization have been prior to your arrival. Consider asking for the past six months' worth of meeting minutes for the teams, committees, or task forces you'll likely participate in. Identify the evolution of the teams, their objectives, and their current status. In addition, become familiar with any legal agreements that you will be accountable for (e.g., vendor, purchasing, employment, consulting, or payer contracts; real estate or equipment leases; financing notes).

PERSONNEL ORIENTATION

Get to know your constituents. To whom do you report? Who reports to you, directly and indirectly? Who are your peers—those on the same managerial or executive level as you? What is the chain of command? An effective leader has a strong rapport with his or her team members, and getting to know them is the first step toward being an effective leader and manager. Once you identify the key players on your team, schedule introductory meetings. Get to know your people and their processes. Ask a lot of questions, and truly listen to the answers. And take a lot of notes.

Perhaps the most important task during your first 90 days is intentional relationship building with your boss. A Gallup survey showed that up to 70 percent of variance in employee engagement is attributable not to compensation, title, rank, office size, or company perks (though all are obviously important) but rather to rapport with one's direct supervisor (Harter and Adkins 2015).

So strive to get to know your leader—his or her leadership style, communication preferences, and personality. Gain as much clarity as possible on your boss's expectations for your performance, the scope of your role, key priorities, and tactical goals for your team or department. Confirm how your effectiveness and success in your role will be measured.

Similarly, if you lead others, invest time in getting to know them, and allow them to get to know you. That rapport will enhance their ability to collaborate positively with their new leader (you) and to engage in their work roles. Earmark this practice as one to repeat throughout your career.

LEARN FROM THOSE AROUND YOU

As you continue on your career path and settle into your leadership style, observe the leaders you admire and how they interact with their teams. What kind of relationship do they have with their teams? How do they communicate with team members? How do they interact with, motivate, or direct their subordinates? How do they navigate conflict or political situations? Take note of what makes a leader a great teammate. Also, with respect and tact, take note of what areas the leaders might improve on when it comes to interacting with their team.

As we've mentioned in other chapters of this book (chapters 1, 9, and 10, to be specific), the most successful leaders are self-aware at every stage of their career. They consistently seek feedback about their performance and engage with mentors and other trusted accountability partners to curate their continued growth and development. This begins on day one! During your first few weeks at your job, request feedback daily from the leaders around you. Throughout your first 90 days, meet frequently with your direct supervisor and any other leaders with whom you will regularly work to solicit their thoughts on your performance so far.

PERSONAL CONSIDERATIONS FOR A NEW JOB

We've talked a lot about the professional considerations of a new job—the people, the organization, the structure, and so on—but what about the personal considerations? A new job often implies a lot of change.

You might be working in a different part of town than you were in your previous job. You might even be in an entirely new city or a new state. Don't let your professional focus overshadow the significant changes happening in your personal life, too.

Ask existing friends and colleagues if they know anyone in your new area and can introduce you. The more connections, the better, for both personal and professional reasons. You might know someone who knows someone who has experience in your industry in your local area. You may know someone who knows someone who has the dish on the best places to eat in town. It's all important!

Begin to familiarize yourself with your new community. Research local chamber groups. Consider checking out nonprofit organizations that might be closely aligned with your professional or personal passions. Have fun exploring the community's history, landmarks, and culture. And be certain to observe your organization's place in the community. How is it perceived? How ingrained is it, or not, in the local community? Does the organization's external brand identity align with your early impressions of its internal cultural identity?

Embrace the change inherent in any new job and intentionally immerse yourself in the new community and organization, but be sure to pace yourself.

WINNING EARLY

Early wins excite and energize people, and they can add to your worth as an important and valued team member. They can win others over and show that you're motivated to make positive contributions as a leader. What are some easy, early successes that a newly onboarding professional can seek in the first three to six months in a role or organization? Here are a few ways that you can make a positive first impression.

1. *Manners matter.* Professional decorum is a strong tell of one's character. Whether you're an intern, an administrative fellow, an analyst, a director, or a senior leader in the organization, being prompt and respecting others' time, saying please and thank you, and following up are critical. Displaying good manners is one of the easiest ways to start building credibility.

2. *Show initiative.* It will naturally take a bit of time to learn about the organization and get your arms around your new role, but individuals who show initiative in

seeking out the conversations that will equip them with knowledge will more quickly establish rapport with everyone around them.

3. *Demonstrate resourcefulness.* Be creative! Through research or networking, put in a little extra legwork to seek out options to bring to the table. Was there a case study in your graduate program that is applicable to a current problem in your new organization? Pull it off the shelf, dust it off, and share it with your team. Did you read an article on Twitter about a creative solution in another industry? Raise your hand and offer it for consideration.

4. *Establish relationships at a variety of levels and departments.* Be approachable. It's prudent in the early stages of onboarding in a role, and no less thereafter, to be visible and engage with folks at every level of your organization. Make time to round in your department and perhaps throughout the organization, on a routine basis. Consider dining in the cafeteria or dropping by the staff lounge, and strike up conversations with those you would not otherwise interact with. And be as mindful of your "social game" as you are of your professional performance. They can both make or break a leader's career.

5. *Demonstrate a strong work ethic.* People are getting to know you, just as you are getting to know them. While first impressions are being formed (and always), it behooves you to show evidence of a strong work ethic. Don't miss deadlines. Underpromise and overdeliver. And be a reliable colleague.

Concrete can easily be formed and augmented when it is first poured, but once it has set, it is permanent and nearly impossible to change. Reputations are the same. Ensure that your first impressions and first contributions are positive ones.

GAINING COMPETENCY

Of course, it goes without saying that you need to be able to perform your new job. Remember the adage "Measure twice, cut once." Make sure that you have a clear understanding of the expectations of your position before you begin. Expectations should be the most important topic of discussion when you first meet with your new boss. Be certain that you have a full grasp of what success will look like, then attack your new work with completeness and accuracy.

Continue to ask questions, but be strategic about doing so. Do not pepper your boss with a barrage of inquiries throughout each day; save them for one meeting, if possible. Try compiling them into an efficient, intelligent list, perhaps even organized into categories. Keep in mind that your boss is busy, so unless you absolutely need to have a question answered immediately, wait until you have a regularly scheduled meeting with him or her.

Do research and ask others who have been, or are currently in, your position. People are usually willing to help, especially at first. Take advantage of all the help you can get. The faster you understand the expectations, freedoms, and limits of your new job, the better.

THE BURDEN OF YOUTH

Many young leaders who are fresh out of school and thrust into the realm of leadership make the mistake of confusing education with experience. There's a good chance that many of the people you will be leading will be older than you. They may have many years of experience in their jobs and have worked for good managers and bad managers.

Good leaders respect their employees and listen to them. We cannot emphasize enough that new leaders must exercise extreme humility. While many managerial decisions ultimately will lie with you, a wise leader seeks counsel from those who have been there before. Those people may include a colleague or boss, but good leaders also often consult frontline staff.

A staff nurse in your department might have an associate's degree. Having a master's degree does not mean you're more intelligent than he is. Nor does it mean that you're better able to contribute value to the organization. Eliciting the help of your team shows your employees that you respect and value their input and that you aren't the type of leader who moves forward blindly without gathering information from many sources.

COMMON PITFALLS TO AVOID

Pace yourself! You're excited and ready to work, but be cautious. Let's look at a few common ways you might make things more difficult for yourself as you get up and running during your first 90 days. (Even beyond 90 days, think of it as a marathon, not a sprint to succeed.)

- *Trying to be everyone's friend.* Use prudence in being warm and personable and in building rapport with your peers and direct reports as you onboard. Be careful about respecting organizational cultural norms and lines of authority.

  Suppose you are a new leader who has become familiar and comfortable with your direct reports. If you must recommend or implement a new process or change that is unpopular, or if you have to enact a budget restriction or cost reduction, your team will quickly become frustrated with your incongruent behavior. Be aware of the fine line between being friendly and being friends.

  Don't get too personal too fast. A naive leader can be eager to make connections, be liked, and become known. Take it easy, tiger! Govern your enthusiasm (remember our discussions about self-awareness?) and use discretion when disclosing facets of your personal life, lest you overshare.

- *Making changes too quickly.* Seasoned executives often come into a new organization and clean house. An emerging leader, eager for an early win as described above, might be tempted to do the same.

  Change is hard for most people and can even be traumatic in some organizational cultures. Early careerists and young leaders should be judicious in recommending and implementing changes, especially at first. Be slow to commit and cautious of any change you think you want to make.

  Keep in mind that a new employee or a new leader can be a target. Some employees might try to test you. Peers may try to dump duties or committee assignments on you, and problem employees may seek to get a new manager to change a policy or bend to their preference. In the first 90 days, resolve not to make long-term changes too quickly. Don't be taken advantage of, and be sure to gain the clarity and context that is required to make sound decisions.

  Early in your career, you should be like a sponge, listening and absorbing as much information as possible, so that by the time you do make changes, your decisions are informed.

- *Not listening before you speak.* You will naturally feel the need to prove yourself early on. Be careful not to form an opinion or speak out of turn before you know what you're talking about or have all the facts. You still have a lot to learn. Listening is a skill, and this is a great time to hone it. You have two ears and one mouth; think about that proportion, and listen and speak accordingly.

- *Always mentioning your previous organization.* It probably goes without saying for a professional, emerging leader such as yourself, but when a newbie incessantly says, "The way we did it at XYZ Health System," others might be insulted or, at a minimum, annoyed. Mentioning your former employer is a natural thing to do—we get it! But just don't do it.
- *Telling people how smart and experienced you are.* Ugh! Don't tell them—show them! Actions speak louder than words. So take a deep breath. You have the education and were hired for this job for a reason. No one expects you to be a pro on day one.

Remember These

- You only have one chance to make a first impression.
- Making mistakes in the first 90 days can be much more harmful than making the same mistakes 6 or 12 months into the job.
- Before your fresh perspective as a newcomer fades, leverage that lens to observe and become familiar with your new organization's culture.
- Perhaps your most important task during your first 90 days is intentional relationship building with your boss. Strive to get to know your leader—his or her leadership style, communication style, personality, and preferences. Gain as much clarity as possible on your boss's expectations for your performance, the scope of your role, key priorities, and tactical goals for your team or department.
- As you continue on your career path and settle into your leadership style, observe the leaders you admire and how they interact with their teams.

→

- Early wins excite and energize people, and they can add to your worth as an important and valued team member. They can win others over and show that you're motivated to make positive contributions as a leader.

- Familiarize yourself with your new community. Embrace the change inherent in any new job and intentionally immerse yourself in the new community and organization, but be sure to pace yourself.

- You're excited and ready to work, but use caution. Avoid common pitfalls, and think of your first 90 days as a marathon, not a sprint.

REFERENCE

Harter, J., and A. Adkins. 2015. "Employees Want a Lot More from Their Managers." *Gallup News*. Published April 8. www.gallup.com/businessjournal/182321/employees-lot-managers.aspx.

Note to My 25-Year-Old Self

Start planning your career when you begin your first position. A sailor has a map to chart the course. Your career deserves the same care—otherwise any road you take will get you only to "a destination."

Begin your journey. Be flexible and open to opportunities that are aligned with your career goals. Don't be rigid about position titles and roles; adapt to the organization's needs. Understand your strengths as well as those areas that require more development. Seek a mentor early on, and use failures and missteps as opportunities to learn. And be vulnerable. In short, it will heighten your self-awareness.

Be yourself. Capitalize on the attributes that come naturally to you. What works for others may not work for you. Approach your projects and work with others in a collaborative manner to assist in achieving organizational objectives. Observe leaders and other professionals regardless of their position. Take notes. Ask questions. Learn, and adopt habits or behaviors that allow you to realize and maximize your full potential. Remember, be humble and you will learn what not to do.

Enter your profession. Consider the skills and knowledge you will gain, not the salary you have been offered. At this stage, you should focus on roles that are the best fit for you and that allow you to bring value to the organization. Honor your commitments and produce results; with results come future opportunities.

Engage in both professional and personal networking, and build relationships. No matter how busy you are, networking is critical. People in your professional network recommend other professionals they know. Membership in professional organizations is an excellent way to cultivate those relationships. On the personal side, sustain family relationships and friendships to achieve work–life balance while maintaining your health, spirituality, and involvement in civic activities. Surround yourself with friends who have the same values as you, and have some fun.

Signed,

Andrea R. Price, FACHE

Governor (2003–2006 and 2013–2016), American College of Healthcare Executives

Strategic Advisor and Consultant, RMP Group LLC

CHAPTER 15

Own and Manage Your Career Path

*I want to look back on my career and be proud of the work,
be proud that I tried everything.*

—*Jon Stewart, former host,* The Daily Show

Reading Points

- Don't Underestimate the Value of an Entry-Level Job
- Do Make It Happen
- Don't Get Comfortable
- Do Chart a Career Path
- Do Act *As If*
- Do Stand Out
- Do Make the Boss Look Good
- Do Win Employees Over, Especially Those Older Than You

EVERY STEP YOU take toward being an accomplished healthcare leader is important. Every step is a learning experience, an opportunity to network and build lasting connections, and an occasion to prepare yourself for the next level and beyond. Take advantage of each step.

Remember what we said way back in chapter 1? Let's remind you: One of the benefits of being self-aware is gaining an intimate knowledge of your character, strengths and weaknesses, and inter-personal style. When you have this understanding, you are in a better position to act. That is, instead of shoehorning yourself into a role simply because it pays well, is prestigious, or is what every-one expects for you, you can chart a career path that suits you best. Doing work that is both meaningful and rewarding is the holy grail for career-minded individuals. That's way more important than any title or pay grade. (Sadly, we know too many well-titled and highly compensated people who are miserable in their jobs.) So get to know yourself; chart a career path; take the initiative to land opportunities, challenge yourself, and stand out; and present your best self and do your best work to stay on your path.

In this chapter, we present the dos and don'ts of managing your career—specifically, at the early stages. Here, we revisit concepts and strategies that we've discussed in earlier chapters. We also provide examples and recommendations taken from real-world experiences.

DON'T UNDERESTIMATE THE VALUE OF AN ENTRY-LEVEL JOB

After completing her undergraduate degree, Laurie took a job as an administrative assistant for the clinic network of a large health system. A glamorous role? Definitely not. A high-paying posi-tion? Hardly. At the time, she was pursuing her master's degree in healthcare administration full-time and was chomping at the bit to move on. She wanted more. She felt like she was not undertaking worthwhile work, and she couldn't wait to realize her potential. (See chapter 9 for another facet of this story.)

In hindsight, Laurie recognizes that the two years she spent in that role taught her things she couldn't have gleaned from a textbook, a case study, or a classroom lecture. She saw how physician practices *really* operated, how every role in the practice functioned, what the physicians did day to day, what their needs and priorities were, how they related to and viewed healthcare administrators, how they interacted with each other and with staff, and what cultural dynamics they stimulated.

That entry-level position was a fertile ground for learning, although Laurie didn't realize it at the time. It prepared her for her subsequent roles, including as a consultant to physician groups.

Our point here is simple: Out of the most unassuming jobs sometimes come rich experiences. If you keep an open mind and embrace these opportunities, instead of taking them for granted, you'll find yourself pleasantly surprised by the career lessons and insights they offer.

No matter what position you hold today and no matter how you feel about it, you must give it the respect it deserves. Make the most of it (more on this later in the chapter) and be grateful for the opportunity. Show up and be stellar at your job every day.

DO MAKE IT HAPPEN

It is whatever you want it to be—a promotion, a C-suite or senior management position, a higher salary, a coveted project, and so on. Don't just sit around and wait for the perfect position, the perfect project, or the perfect salary. Keep your eyes open for new or additional opportunities. Volunteer. Identify a need and fill it. Choose a problem and solve it. Define what you want, be prepared to do the work involved, and ask for the opportunity to pursue it. Be specific, and be certain that you have the time to invest.

Making something happen is about taking the initiative, about taking the reins of your career path. Following are examples of how two professionals made the big leaps happen early on in their careers.

John's Story

John started his banking career at the bottom of the corporate ladder. He was so low on the rung, he joked, that he wasn't sure if he was even on the ladder at all! His title sounded nice enough—junior analyst—but the job was the very definition of entry level. His desk was right next to the copy machine, which was convenient, as copying was among his foremost responsibilities.

Unsatisfied with his job, John began to look around himself—literally. He noticed a stack of dusty banker's boxes in the office. They contained old, forgotten collection files. He approached his supervisors and asked if he could sift through the boxes and address the accounts. He got the go-ahead.

Slowly but surely, John dug in and reconciled each account. His work led to the bank recouping money owed; these were dollars that would have remained in boxes had he not volunteered to revisit the accounts. His initiative, his willingness to do the grunt work everyone else avoided, and his strong work ethic that made him go above and beyond his expected duties resulted in his advancement to collector and then loan officer. He spent a decade as a vice president, and today he is a bank president.

Mallory's Story

Mallory is an emerging leader in healthcare. Her story perfectly illustrates how taking the initiative can move you many steps forward on your career path. Here she is in her own words:

> I introduced myself to the CEO after my graduate class took a Level 1 trauma tour of his facility. I told him I grew up in a neighboring county and always admired the mission of the organization. I told him I knew the excellent work he was doing to change the culture here, and I would love to discuss any opportunity to complete an administrative internship to learn from him and his team. He scheduled a meeting, and we discussed that the organization did

not have a formal internship program. After some discussion, he offered me an opportunity to help build a program that summer.

The internship structure began with biweekly meetings with the CEO and COO [chief operating officer] so that I could consistently communicate with and learn from them. We built a schedule where I spent a couple of weeks with each VP [vice president] and their direct reports, holding introductory meetings, taking tours, and attending department meetings. My rotations covered departments such as operations, nursing, medical staff, quality, community health, and IT [information technology]. I also attended all executive and board meetings. I worked on different projects for the VPs. There was not a closed door, which made for a great learning environment.

At the end of the summer, we mutually agreed to extend the internship through my second year of MHA studies. My role was redefined to focus on more in-depth projects in finance and IT. I worked on many projects with the CFO [chief financial officer]. I continued to attend senior-level meetings and board meetings, and I prepared reports for some senior meetings. I continued to serve on the quarterly leadership institute planning committee (and I still do today). I spent some time in planning meetings and steering committees but had no direct responsibility. I continued to work with the CFO on projects and enjoyed his leadership and teaching style immensely.

During my internship, I was supposed to focus mainly on finance and community health, along with other small responsibilities in various other areas. But community health had new leadership, and I was struggling with gaining traction in projects there. When I told the CFO I had more time to give him, he assigned me to the waiver program, giving me a more visible role in the community and exposing me to new experiences. My life changed overnight. The waiver program has been an incredible career opportunity. It has contributed to my success in my role.

DON'T GET COMFORTABLE

When you get comfortable, you stop trying new approaches and stop stretching past your comfort zone. And you wait for, not seek, challenges that keep you on your toes, keep your adrenaline pumping, or get your heart racing. But those who achieve greatness rarely wait. Instead, they hunt, fully knowing that any short-term discomfort from such challenges is a small price to pay for long-term success.

What are these challenges? They could be anything from adopting a bold strategy to setting (and achieving) stretch goals to defying conventions. The idea is to take a risk and to try new things, even if it means failing, so that you can learn and grow.

Early in her career, Natalie applied for jobs for which she wasn't *fully* qualified (see chapter 9 for another facet of this story). For example, if the job posting called for seven to ten years' experience and she only had three to five years under her belt, it didn't stop her from applying. Of course, she met all the other qualifications and could back up her application with references, a record of solid work performance, and relevant skills and training. And of course, she disclosed her lack of years of experience. But she took calculated risks to at least be seen and be considered and at best be given a chance to prove herself. She was stretching, reaching to get her foot in the door.

This strategy not only opened doors but also allowed her to skip multiple rungs on the proverbial career ladder. This example may especially resonate with fresh-out-of-school careerists trying to land their first job but running straight into a requirement they can't fill yet. It's a problem faced by generation after generation of job seekers: Every hiring organization wants a certain amount of on-the-job experience. But young applicants can't meet that qualification if they are not given the opportunity to gain the experience required.

Don't get lulled by the routine of your job. Teach yourself a new skill while you're at it. While in school, Natalie used to work at a chain clothing store at the mall. She knew she wasn't going to work there forever, so she focused on developing new skills. Not only did she get good at anticipating and meeting the needs of the customers, but she also learned how to input data via ten-key. When the store wasn't busy, she rang up purchases by typing SKU (stock-keeping unit) numbers into the system rather than scanning the item tags. She timed herself each time and got better and better. Before too long she had mastered the skill and was just as fast manually entering the SKU numbers as scanning them. She still uses the ten-key skill today, not to mention the customer service skills she developed.

Whatever you do, get into the habit of challenging and stretching yourself. Don't simply float along. Make some waves.

DO CHART A CAREER PATH

Put pen to paper and write out a path or plan for your career. Make it specific, manage or keep an eye on it, measure your progress against it, and modify it when needed. Most important, stick to it.

Not many things go exactly as planned (Laurie's nonlinear career path is a perfect example), but nothing goes anywhere (only round and round in a circle perhaps) without a plan. We can't promise that your career path will lead you to your desired destination, but we can guarantee that just by charting a path, you're already ahead of the others who don't or won't take the time to sit down and write a plan.

If you need help charting this path or are unclear about what a healthcare career path looks like, consult your mentor or a seasoned administrator or even your own boss. Don't hesitate to interview leaders in your organization or the industry (you can meet them when you attend national events like the American College of Healthcare Executives Congress on Healthcare Leadership). Start a conversation: So, you're a chief strategy officer, what does that entail? What projects are you involved in right now? How does your job relate to the rest of the organization? Be a student of your profession. Then, use that knowledge to chart your own path.

Now here are the *buts*:

- *But you have to be a doer.* Charting a path—even if it's color coded, laminated, animated, graphic designed, and Instagrammed—is not enough. You have to do the hard work. The path is merely a guideline and isn't going to walk itself.
- *But you have to be realistic.* You can accelerate the timing of your plan goals all you want, but be prepared for disappointment when you don't hit those time frames. Manage your own expectations. Know that you're going to have to apply some elbow grease and pay your dues. The leaders and other healthcare professionals before you poured blood, sweat, and tears into their paths. Expect to do the same. Make room for failures, mistakes, and rejections (see chapter 9). Setbacks are learning opportunities, but they can unexpectedly derail your path. They will happen, but you can't schedule them.

DO ACT *AS IF*

This goes back to our personal brand discussion in chapter 6. Carry yourself *as if* you are already in the position you aspire to have. We're talking character-based conduct here, not inflated ego. When you act *as if*, you're likely to make a positive impression and to be regarded as someone who is ready or at least has the potential for the next level. Plus, when you act *as if* and back that up with your strengths (including self-awareness, strong character, and commitment and self-discipline), people will see you as indispensable. You'll be that person everyone thinks they can't do without, that person whom everyone hates to see go at the end of the day. (As Natalie's mom advised her: "Work in such a way that when it's time to go, they hate to see you leave.")

Dress the Part

Top-notch leaders don't just act like top-notch leaders, they look like them, too. Again, dress *as if.* If your role calls for business casual attire, press the envelope and wear the sharpest business attire (if the organizational culture and situation allow, of course). Invest in a power suit—that one tailored piece that makes you feel more confident, taller, and brighter. Polish your shoes. And let your smile be your best accessory. You'll be amazed at how good dressing well makes you feel and how differently others treat you.

Be Authentic

We understand that sometimes when people hear "acting/dressing *as if,*" they immediately think that only those who present themselves in such a way can succeed. Not true, and not what we're saying. Figure out who you are first (again, practice self-reflection). Then, conduct and dress yourself according to the true you. Do polish yourself, because the more put-together you look, the more you and what you have to offer shine and the less likely your appearance will serve as a distraction. You don't have to wear designer clothes or trendy pieces (who has the budget for that?!), but you do have to follow the organization's dress code or standard professional clothing.

The more important thing to remember is to be authentic. Don't dress, act, or talk exactly like someone else; that person is already taken. You do you—the best version of you. If you don't, you will at some point find yourself miserable and others will think you're a fraud.

With the combination of good attitude and good look, you'll feel different—as if you can go anywhere and accomplish anything. You can transform a job you feel is not the right fit for you into one that is a beneficial learning opportunity. The job itself remains the same. It's your mind-set that changes.

DO STAND OUT

You may not want to be in your current position for the rest of your life, but are you actively doing something about it? For many, the path to the next level often seems littered with obstacles and delays. You yearn to run but feel fenced in. You're revving your engine, but the light hasn't turned green. We know; we've been there.

One of the surest ways to get a chance, a break, or a yes is to be a contributor. Organizations—healthcare facilities included—are filled with people who don't want to step up. They are filled with critics and cynics and standbys. So people like you—with skills and talents and ambition—are certainly wanted and needed. Take the initiative (see John's and Mallory's stories earlier in the chapter) and stand up and stand out.

Know your strengths. What can you do that no one else can? What can you do better and faster and longer than anyone else can? Is there a need that's not obvious but has to be filled anyway? Can you create a need for what you can do? For example, you could volunteer to take the minutes for a senior management meeting (a meeting you might otherwise not be invited to). If you don't show up one day, people will start looking for you. Just by showing up all the time and being the person who does something, you've planted a seed that you're *supposed* to be there, that you belong. And people may need you for other projects—big and small.

DO MAKE THE BOSS LOOK GOOD

It may be tough to overcome the stigma attached to the notion of "making the boss look good." After all, nobody wants to be labeled a suck-up. It's certainly a delicate situation. On one hand, you want to endear yourself to the boss. On the other hand, you don't want to be alienated from the rest of the team.

Think of it this way: You need to look out for what is best for you and your career. If that means making the boss look good by doing a great job, so be it. Plenty of your peers want the role and responsibilities you'll possibly land by taking the initiative to work closely with the boss, but they're either too afraid to pursue the opportunity or they don't want to put in the extra work. If they ostracize you because of that, then that's on them, not you.

Now, let's be very clear on one thing: We aren't giving you permission to be a suck-up! We're simply encouraging you to be a key contributor, to be that go-to person, to pay your dues.

One of Laurie's organization clients has a term for people who don't want to get involved when they see a problem: *short-arm syndrome*. It describes those who pull their arms back, palms facing outward, and say, "Hey, that's not my job!" The opposite of short-arm syndrome is represented by those who are ready and willing to help, to take responsibility, and to be the go-to person. A little dirt under your fingernails, so to speak, is a badge of honor! Go for it. Extend those arms to the boss.

Why Do It?

1. *It demonstrates your promotion worthiness or potential.*
   Let's face it, managers initiate most career advances for their staff. Knocking the supervisor's socks off may mean a little more cash in your pocket, a nice reference or recommendation or write-up in your employee file, or even a promotion offer. You may not be a senior team member now, but if you consistently prove yourself to be an ace, your boss may start to visualize you as an individual worthy of promotion.

2. *It instills humility in you.* Looking out for another person solidifies that you're a member of the team, which is something bigger than yourself.

3. *It gives you valuable in-the-trenches experience.* Often, focusing on your boss and making her look good takes you outside of your day-to-day responsibilities. Not only do you earn brownie points with the boss, but you also garner new experiences you would not have had at your desk.

How Should I Do It?

1. *Go above and beyond.* It's not enough to do (and do well) what's expected of you. You have to also volunteer to do tasks that are not in your job description, that just came up, or that no one else wants to do. And you have to give your best work, not half-baked attempts or bare minimums just to get it over with. Find ways to show you are willing to take on and complete these extra tasks. Be so good that you convince everyone you are indispensable.

2. *Share your strengths.* Master organizer and coordinator? IT genius? Superb troubleshooter, writer, negotiator? Charmer? Customer service maven? Finance expert? Whatever your thing, let it be known. This isn't bragging about what you can do. This is informing those who need to know that you're available to help in specific areas when needed.

3. *Offer solutions.* Organizations are fraught with people who like to complain about everything that's wrong. Instead of jumping on that bandwagon, dare to be different by offering workable solutions to those problems. Leverage your skills, talents, and energy to take the initiative and improve your organization, as opposed to adding to the problem or maintaining the status quo.

DO WIN EMPLOYEES OVER, ESPECIALLY THOSE OLDER THAN YOU

Winning people over is a matter of trust. Establishing trust means you're in it for the long haul, not a quick sprint. It's not easy, but then again, nothing worth having is. In healthcare, it is incredibly common for your employees to be older than you—often by several decades. After all, four generations of workers serve in healthcare facilities, and many clinical and administrative positions are held by seasoned professionals.

Many challenges come with this younger boss–older employee dynamic. We both have experienced this, and we still do. Laurie, in particular, was responsible for managing more than three dozen employees when she was only 22. Every one of them was older; one nurse's date of hire was in the same year Laurie was born. She heard comments such as, "I wonder how long till blondie gets chewed up and spit out!" and "I've watched so many managers come and go, and when you leave I will still be here."

As an emerging healthcare leader, you have to be prepared for this eventuality. Exhibit 15.1 offers tips for establishing rapport with your employees despite the generation gaps.

Exhibit 15.1 Tips for Managing Employees Older Than You

1. *Treat all employees with genuine respect.* Your character and conduct trump almost all your other accomplishments. If employees see that you sincerely care about their roles and needs, they won't see your age. Your date of birth will be ignored and your qualities as a person and as a leader will shine. As the saying goes, "People don't care how much you know until they know how much you care."
2. *Listen.* Get in the habit of seeking out conversations with all employees, communicating often with members of your teams and departments. The more you get to know your staff through these conversations, the better you'll be able to provide resources. And the more you know people—their talents, abilities, and contributions—the more effectively you can engage, inspire, and acknowledge them.

(continued)

3. *Lead by example.* Set the tone by exhibiting the integrity, work ethic, and attitude you hope to see in your team. Twenty-somethings often get a bad reputation for feeling entitled. If your contributions and conduct are strong, they'll speak for you. Show up early, stay late, and be a team player.

4. *Show humility.* Acknowledge the value of others, and generously give credit where credit is due. Don't be afraid to say, "I don't know the answer, but I will find out." There is no better way than that to prove your humility or to build rapport and trust with your employees—especially those who might have issues with the age gap. As you grow into your career, be humble about the fact that no one—not even you—can know everything all the time. There are too many moving parts in healthcare. But everyone is an expert in their respective areas. The hospital's compliance officer, for example, may know the ins and outs of Joint Commission accreditation better than he knows himself, but he may be at a loss when asked about Clinical Laboratory Improvement Amendments (CLIA) waiver certification for the laboratory or what the oncology floor requires for its intravenous competencies.

5. *Learn from the wise.* You will always have smart people around you from whom you can learn (e.g., your board of career advisors). They are individuals whose experiences and expertise far outweigh yours. As a leader, your role isn't to be the utmost authority on all matters but to strategically align resources with organizational goals. Glean wisdom from those who have been around longer than you have. If they've been there, done that—especially for a long time within the current organization—don't hesitate to leverage that experience. Kindly, of course. Doing so could equip you with valuable insight. Learn from their mistakes and lessons learned.

Remember These

- Out of the most unassuming jobs sometimes come rich experiences. If you keep an open mind and embrace these opportunities instead of taking them for granted, you'll find yourself pleasantly surprised by the career lessons and insights they offer.

- Keep your eyes open for new or additional opportunities. Volunteer. Identify a need and fill it.

→

Choose a problem and solve it. Define what you want, be prepared to do the work involved, and ask for the opportunity to pursue it.

- Don't get lulled by the routine of your job. Teach yourself a new skill while you're at it.

- Make your boss look good by being his or her go-to person or key contributor. Knocking the supervisor's socks off just may mean a little more cash in your pocket, a nice reference or recommendation or write-up in your employee file, or even a promotion offer.

- For emerging healthcare leaders, it is incredibly common for your employees to be older than you—often by several decades. Your character and conduct trump almost all your other accomplishments. If employees see that you sincerely care about their roles and needs, they won't care about the generation gap.

Books That Teach, Advise, and Inspire Us

Laurie's List

1. *The Advantage: Why Organizational Health Trumps Everything Else in Business* by Patrick Lencioni
2. *Mindset: The New Psychology of Success* by Carol S. Dweck
3. *Essentialism: The Disciplined Pursuit of Less* by Greg McKeown
4. *Emotional Intelligence: Why It Can Matter More Than IQ* by Daniel Goleman
5. *The Power of Habit: Why We Do What We Do* by Charles Duhigg
6. *Strengths Based Leadership: Great Leaders, Teams, and Why People Follow* by Tom Rath and Barry Conchie
7. *The Speed of Trust: The One Thing That Changes Everything* by Stephen M. R. Covey
8. *Wooden on Leadership: How to Create a Winning Organization* by John Wooden and Steve Jamison
9. *Daring Greatly: How the Courage to Be Vulnerable Transforms the Way We Live, Love, Parent, and Lead* by Brené Brown
10. *Failing Forward: Turning Mistakes into Stepping Stones for Success* by John C. Maxwell
11. *Executive Excellence: Protocols for Healthcare Leaders*, 2nd ed., by Carson F. Dye

12. *Grit: The Power of Passion and Perseverance* by Angela Duckworth

13. *Originals: How Non-Conformists Move the World* by Adam Grant

Natalie's List

1. *How to Win Friends and Influence People* by Dale Carnegie

2. *Management Lessons from Mayo Clinic: Inside One of the World's Most Admired Service Organizations* by Leonard L. Berry and Kent D. Seltman

3. *Over Our Heads: An Analogy on Healthcare, Good Intentions, and Unforeseen Consequences* by Rulon F. Stacey

4. *The One Minute Manager* by Kenneth H. Blanchard and Spencer Johnson

5. *Developing the Leader Within You* by John C. Maxwell

6. *HBR's 10 Must Reads: On Leadership, On Managing People, On Managing Yourself* (compilation of articles)

7. *Executive Charisma: Six Steps to Mastering the Art of Leadership* by D. A. Benton

8. *Good to Great: Why Some Companies Make the Leap . . . and Others Don't* by Jim Collins

9. *The Effective Executive: The Definitive Guide to Getting the Right Things Done* by Peter F. Drucker

10. *The Practice of Management* by Peter F. Drucker

11. *The Servant: A Simple Story About the True Essence of Leadership* by James C. Hunter

12. *Fierce Conversations: Achieving Success at Work and in Life One Conversation at a Time* by Susan Scott

13. *Execution: The Discipline of Getting Things Done* by Larry Bossidy and Ram Charan

Frequently Asked Questions
(and Our Answers)

When we mentor and interact with graduate students and emerging healthcare leaders, we consistently hear a few of the same questions. Here they are, with our answers.

What skills will make me stand out early in my career?

First, soft skills are just as important as technical skills. As discussed in chapters 1 and 3 and in examples throughout the book, the ability to build relationships, read situations, and practice active listening is essential to your success in an organization. For example, the ability to have a crucial conversation about the budget with your employees is just as important as being able to perform a financial analysis. As an early careerist, possessing emotional intelligence can help catapult you through the ranks. Are you self-reflective? Are you aware of your blind spots and do you actively manage how you are perceived? Do you pick up social cues well? Can you have a fluid, meaningful conversation and garner important information that helps you understand and better communicate with your constituents? If not, work on these competencies. Such skills will set you apart from the rest. Some things we just have to experience and learn, but if you can observe and skip the experience part (especially the painful experiences), that too will set you apart.

Should I pursue a fellowship or go straight into a job? Will one or the other set me up for greater success?

There is no right answer to this question. It depends on what you are trying to accomplish and what type of experience you want to gain. Entering a fellowship and going straight into the real world of work each has its pros and cons. A fellowship can propel you a few years ahead of where you would be if you headed straight into a new career in healthcare. When you finish your fellowship program, you'll likely be placed in a role significantly higher than an entry-level position because of the depth and breadth of your experiences during your fellowship year. In addition, you will nurture relationships and have the opportunity to participate in significant projects, allowing you to harness new skills. However, a fellowship might not be an option for you because of your career path preference, target organization or organization type, or a geographic restriction. Fear not—many emerging leaders transition directly from their academic programs into the workplace and successfully navigate their career and leadership growth journey. Our advice is to seek as many conversations as possible within your network regarding opportunities and experiences, and compare your findings to your goals and circumstances.

If pursuing a fellowship is not an option, what types of jobs and experiences should I look for?

Emerging healthcare leaders have a wide array of organizations and roles to consider. Organization types include academic medical centers, integrated health systems, critical access hospitals, behavioral healthcare organizations, payer organizations, and consulting firms, to name a few. The diversity in roles includes operational management, finance, analysis, strategy, health policy, community health, organizational development, project management, and many more. The best advice, for both the early stages of your career and consistently thereafter, is to carefully consider your strengths and weaknesses, your skill set, and your key purpose and motivation. Pursuing a specific role or organization purely because it is considered the "holy grail" in the industry is a sure recipe for disaster. If 80 percent of the students in your graduate program class covet the hospital C-suite as their ultimate career path destination but you yearn for strategy and innovation, follow your gut. Too many climb the ladder to "success" only to realize that it's leaning against the wrong building.

With a push for more clinicians to fill healthcare leadership roles, what can I, an individual from a nonclinical background, do to stay competitive?

It always behooves you to know your industry well. You must strive to be a resident expert at your work. If you are not clinically trained, being able to speak the language of the clinician is extremely helpful. Not only does it boost your credibility, but it also helps you understand how your work influences the clinical side. Buy a general medical terms textbook. Look up common procedures performed in the department you work in. Shadow a physician or nurse to better understand the operational portion of the practice of medicine: initial exam, tests, notes/dictations, and so on. There is no better way to understand the ins and outs of the clinical side than by seeing them firsthand. If the situation presents itself, sit down and interview a practitioner. Not only will this bolster your relationship with that individual by generating rapport and showing a genuine interest in his or her work, it will also help you cultivate important medical vocabulary. Work on being a lifelong learner. Read, read, and read some more.

How should I approach networking when I'm no longer a graduate student and in the early years of my career?

Networking when you're a student can be easier than when you've started your career in the industry. Because they remember when they were students and sought guidance, most healthcare leaders are more than willing to help students and offer their time for mentoring and shadowing programs. However, once you depart academia and begin your healthcare leadership career, you become a peer to people in the industry. You have a new opportunity to establish yourself in an organization, a community, a geographic region. Seek to build new connections. Become acquainted with those who are well regarded by others in the organization, and work diligently to establish a personal brand as an individual of strong integrity, work ethic, service mentality, and decorum. Never stop networking and expanding your personal and professional connections. Like compound interest, the earlier and more consistently you make deposits into your network "bank account," the greater dividends it will pay.

Aside from on-the-job experiences, what are the best resources for learning after leaving graduate school?

To be successful in healthcare, you must be a lifelong learner. To keep learning about healthcare, take advantage of traditional resources such as trade magazines, association offerings and websites, podcasts, relevant online healthcare groups, and the like. Professional development will be beneficial throughout your career, but especially early on. Register for webinars and go to conferences or seminars that interest you and that may help you hone a skill or learn about the latest developments in the industry. Always invest the time to read the latest industry publications, to keep your finger on the pulse of what is happening and who is leading work where. And make sure you're "in the room" in your organization and community, and in the healthcare industry, to stay abreast and engaged as time goes on.

Early in my career, how should I approach an assignment on a topic that I have minimal or no experience with?

There are myriad resources at your fingertips to learn about the topic. To equip yourself to complete the assignment, take the initiative to research internal and external resources, including those throughout your network. But also sit down with the person assigning the project and make certain you understand the project's objective and what the work entails. If appropriate, ask about expected outcomes. Make sure that you have adequate access to the organizational resources you may need to get the job done. Finally, ask for candid feedback on your performance, and accept it gracefully. No one expects you to have all the answers, especially early in your career. The best thing you can do is to show up well informed and with a willing spirit, a solid work ethic, and a humble approach. The worst thing you can do is to fail to demonstrate engagement or resourcefulness, to shirk accountability, and to underperform.

I feel like business etiquette has changed over the years, perhaps because of technology. Is it still necessary to be so formal in the workplace?

Some might scoff at the notion of professional etiquette, but we advise that you err on the side of prudence. There is a perception that *traditional* means "out-of-date" or "stodgy and stuffy," but if you take time to learn the rules of engagement, you can avoid making a simple social mistake that may cause others to think you are not a positive representative of the organization. Professional decorum and etiquette—not just a strong resume and academic track record—often make the difference between getting an interview, an internship or fellowship, or the nod to advance in your organization and ending up in the "thank you for applying, but" category. You may have an appetite for risk taking and innovation, and it may serve you well in your tactical performance. But our advice to emerging leaders in healthcare is to play it very close to the line when curating your personal and professional brand. Always wear the suit. Be sharp. Be early. Stay late. Do your research. Engage. Volunteer. Be humble. Send handwritten thank-you notes. Go the extra mile. Forgo that second drink at professional events. Some things go out of style, but manners do not.

About the Authors

Laurie K. Baedke, MHA, FACHE, FACMPE, is a faculty member, the director of healthcare leadership programs, and program director for the Executive MBA in Healthcare Management at Creighton University.

A frequent speaker at national healthcare conferences and facilitator at company and association retreats, Laurie works with teams and individuals including early careerists, physician leaders, and senior executives. She has specific expertise in physician practice management, leadership development, organizational change, emotional intelligence, and strengths-based leadership.

Laurie holds a bachelor's degree in human services and business administration and a master's degree in healthcare administration. She is a Fellow of the American College of Healthcare Executives (ACHE) and of the American College of Medical Practice Executives, as well as a member of the Medical Group Management Association. She has been certified by Gallup as a strengths performance coach since 2006.

Laurie is the recipient of numerous awards, including the Nebraska ACHE Regent's Early Career Excellence Award (2001), the District Five ACHE Regent's Award for Healthcare Excellence (2006), and the ACHE Distinguished Service Award (2015).

Professionally, she has served on three national ACHE committees: the Early Careerist; Programs, Products and Services; and Chapters committees. Currently, she is a member of ACHE's Examination Committee and the ACHE of Nebraska and Western

Iowa Chapter board of directors. She also serves a variety of civic and community organizations, including appointments on the Omaha Bridges Out of Poverty board of directors executive committee and the Leadership Omaha curriculum committee.

Laurie recently contributed a chapter titled "The Clinician Entrepreneur" to *The Handbook of Private Practice* (Oxford University Press, 2017).

Laurie lives just outside of Omaha, Nebraska, with her husband and two children.

Natalie D. Lamberton, MBA/MHA, FACHE, is the CEO of New Health Pain Treatment Centers, a medical home for Medicaid and Medicare beneficiaries. Each center houses its own clinic for physical and psychological evaluations and pain treatment and a state-licensed ambulatory surgery center. Prior to this position, she served as the chief operating officer of Jackson North Medical Center, a 382-bed hospital in North Miami, Florida, and as the CEO of Regency Hospital of Fort Worth, Texas. Her career in healthcare leadership has been extensive. She served as the director of neurosciences at the Medical Center of Aurora; as an administrator in Presbyterian Health System, where she oversaw a $190 million construction project for a new hospital; as CEO of the Haxtun Hospital District, which comprised a hospital, an extended care unit, and three primary care clinics serving communities within a 300-square-mile radius; and as the director of retail services of the Poudre Valley Health System, where she designed, developed, and implemented the corporate strategic plan for the division. In addition, she was the first postgraduate administrative fellow for Poudre Valley.

Natalie is the recipient of several awards. In 2016, she was selected as one of *Legacy* magazine's 50 Most Powerful and Influential Black Leaders of Miami. Other awards include the American College of Healthcare Executives (ACHE) Exemplary Service Award (2014), the ACHE Distinguished Service Award (2013), the ACHE Service Award (2011), and the ACHE Regent's Early Careerist Award (2009), among others.

She has served on numerous committees and boards, including ACHE's ache.org Editorial Board and Health Administration Press's Management Series Editorial Board. She has served as a board member of the ACHE Regent's Advisory Council and on the Colorado Association of Healthcare Executives board for several years, and on several councils and committees of the Colorado Hospital Association. She is a Fellow of ACHE and a member of the National Association of Health Services Executives. Natalie is also an advisory board member for Meridian Health Services Network and its 2018 president.

In addition, Natalie has been a guest lecturer (discussing leadership and management) for Creighton University's Heider College of Business MBA program, the University of Iowa's College of Public Health MHA–MBA program, the University of New Mexico Anderson Executive MBA program, Brigham Young University's Marriott School MPA program, and the University of Texas at Dallas Naveen Jindal School of Management graduate program, among others. Her passion is mentoring and inspiring new leaders.

She earned a bachelor of science degree in molecular biology and US history from the University of New Mexico, graduating cum laude. While there, she ran track and field on a full-ride Division I scholarship. A recipient of the distinguished University of Colorado Hoffman-Binger Graduate Presidential Scholarship, Natalie holds a dual MBA and MHA degree from the University of Colorado at Denver. A former teacher, she taught science and history at the middle school and high school levels; she also was a freshman biology instructor at the Community College of Denver.

Natalie lives in the heart of Denver, Colorado, with her husband.